THE REPUBLIC OF THERAPY

....

Triage and Sovereignty in

....

West Africa's Time of AIDS

....

VINH-KIM NGUYEN

....

Duke University Press

Durham and London   2010

© 2010 Duke University Press

All rights reserved

Printed in the United States of America on acid-free paper ∞

Designed by Heather Hensley

Typeset in Minion Pro by Tseng Information Systems, Inc.

Library of Congress Cataloging-in-Publication Data appear
on the last printed page of this book.

...

THE

REPUBLIC

OF

THERAPY

...

BODY, COMMODITY, TEXT   Studies of Objectifying Practice

... *A series edited by Arjun Appadurai, Jean Comaroff, and Judith Farquhar* ...

To my parents

....

For Jennifer Nguyen

CONTENTS

ACKNOWLEDGMENTS

I first encountered medical anthropology in 1982 while an under-
graduate attending a course taught by Margaret Lock. When the AIDS
epidemic was just beginning, and before I went to medical school,
Margaret encouraged me to think about the social implications of the
epidemic and has continued to do so ever since. James Tully, Darius
Rejali, and Brian Walker showed me how political theory could help
make sense of the world. In medical school and residency, Jean-
François Letendre, Ken Marshall, J. D. MacLean, and Jean Wilkins
taught me the science and the art of clinical medicine. In addition,
Ann Macaulay first showed me the importance of community-based
clinical research.

Once I was in practice, Christos M. Tsoukas encouraged my involvement in HIV care and research long before effective treatments
became available. Mariella Pandolfi and Judith Farquhar persuaded
me to pursue a doctorate and influence me still. This book's many
lives began as a doctoral dissertation under the supervision of Margaret Lock. In London Jeff O'Malley, Erika Dix, and Josef Gardiner
were early partners in an experiment that culminated in the International HIV/AIDS Alliance. Christophe Cornu, Beth Mbaka, Paul
McCarrick, Kevin Orr, and Ioanna Trilivas were mentors, colleagues,
and friends throughout my work with community groups in West
Africa. In Abidjan, Philippe Msellati and Laurent Vidal welcomed me
and afforded me an intellectual home away from home at the Centre ORSTOM de Petit-Bassam. Auguste-Didier Blibolo generously invited me to share an office at the Centre. Early on in the course of my

doctorate, I benefitted from the critical mentorship of Nancy Hunt, who has remained an important interlocutor. A fellowship year at the Wissenschafts-kolleg zu Berlin proved critical to undertaking this book. In Berlin, discussions with Yehuda Elkana, Elisio Macamo, and Sebastian Conrad helped me to clarify central lines of inquiry. Shalini Randeria has proven to be a wise and insightful critic ever since. Support from the Max Planck Institute for Social Anthropology's program on Law, Organization, Science and Technology in Africa proved crucial to finishing the research and writing up the results presented in this book.

In Abidjan and Ouagadougou, I am particularly indebted to the hospitality and generosity of Cyriaque Yapo Ako, Yves Kapfer, Eugène Rayess, Issoufou Tiendrébéogo, Constance Yaï, and Abass Zein. Henri Chenal invited me to come and work with him at the Centre Intégré de Recherches Biocliniques d'Abidjan (CIRBA), and I am indebted to the magnificent team there and particularly Emma and Léontine. Most importantly, I owe a debt to the patients and informants who opened their hearts and their families to me.

This book could not have been written without the continuing support of all my colleagues at the Clinique médicale l'Actuel. Réjean Thomas and Line Provost went out of their way to make it possible for me to continue my work in West Africa while practicing in Montreal. At the Université de Montréal, Marie-France Raynault, Cécile Tremblay, and Maria-Victoria Zunzunegui helped me juggle writing and managing a busy research portfolio. At the Jewish General Hospital's Emergency Department, Bernie Unger and Alex Guttman resolved scheduling issues crucial to freeing up the time to finish this book. Finally, the support of Richard Rottenburg and the Max Planck Institute for Social Anthropology, where I was an associate from 2005 to 2010, provided the intellectual space and research support essential to finishing this project.

This book is enriched by conversations, arguments, and meals shared with a community of scholars—a history that makes the claim of authorship of this book somehow uncomfortable. Over the years, discussions with Sean Brotherton, Alice Desclaux, Jean-Pierre Dozon, Didier Fassin, Margaret Lock, Rob Lorway, Laurence McFalls, Kris Peterson, Bernard Taverne, Bob White, Susan Reynolds-Whyte, and Richard Rottenburg have played an important role in shaping the ideas behind this book. I gratefully acknowledge Martha Cadieux, Ari Gandsman, Anitra Grisales, Stephanie Lloyd, Peter Lock, Frank Runcie, and three anonymous reviewers for critical readings of previous versions of this book. For whatever flaws remain, I take full responsibility.

The research on which this book reports would not have been possible without the generous institutional recognition I have received over the years. In addition to granting me doctoral and postdoctoral fellowships, the Social Science and Humanities Research Council of Canada (SSHRC) also awarded me its Aurora Prize in 2007. I am particularly grateful for the SSHRC's support and also the Canadian Institutes of Health Research for a New Investigator Award. For their forbearance and support, I owe a debt to Ken Wissoker and Duke University Press for seeing this project through.

Writing can seem a solitary business, but, in this case, it has been much more of a family affair. My curiosity about Abidjan stems from my maternal grandmother's description to me, when I was perhaps six-years-old, of her trips to visit my aunt Nicole Kapfer and her family in the African colonies and her misadventures while changing planes some time in the late 1960s in what I heard to be "Habite-Jean."

Nicole has since been a constant inspiration. Her stories of living in West Africa for thirty-five years, where she raised her four children, helped me understand the importance of the kind of history you cannot get from books. I must also acknowledge those in my family who made real for me the struggles whose outcomes we now take for granted. Aunt Marie Claire, whose experiences as a nurse in Tunisia during the Second World War and in postwar Europe taught me that medicine can be a vector for social justice even through the horrors of war. My father's brother, Uncle Khuong, told me stories when I accompanied him on Saturday afternoons on his rounds as a pharmacy messenger about how my paternal grandfather had outwitted the French in Indochina. Last but not least, I acknowledge those who have over the past years made for a loving household: Mai-Linh Nguyen, Massinissa Si Mehand, and, most of all, Frank Runcie.

CÔTE-D'IVOIRE AND TRIAGE

IN THE TIME OF AIDS

In 1994, two years after he found out he was HIV positive, a young Abidjan law student named Dominique Esmel founded one of the first groups of people living with HIV in Africa, Light for AIDS. "We chose that name because we felt we were living in darkness," Dominique told me; "we wanted to come out of the shadows of our isolation and live in the light of solidarity."

At the time, AIDS was already the leading cause of death in many parts of the continent, including in Côte-d'Ivoire's bustling port metropolis, Abidjan.[1] Few knew, or had been told, of their diagnosis — not that it would have made much difference then. HIV testing wasn't readily available, and health care workers were reluctant to disclose a "hopeless" diagnosis. When Dominique "came out" publicly with his HIV diagnosis, the focus of the struggle against the epidemic in Africa had begun to shift away from epidemiological surveillance and public awareness campaigns aimed at increasing condom use. Worried that the campaigns weren't working, international agencies bemoaned what they called a "culture of denial." They emphasized the need to "put a face" to the disease. The number of Africans getting tested for HIV must increase, they insisted. More individuals like Dominique would need to "come out" publicly about being HIV positive. I first began to work in West Africa the same year Dominique testified.

I remember first hearing about a mysterious and terrifying new epidemic, reported in gay men in 1982, in my first year of university.

AIDS, as it came to be called, was both a biological and a political issue. In my molecular biology seminars, we examined the workings of a virus that defied biological orthodoxy by reversing the flow of genetic information in order to integrate itself into the host's genetic material. Reports of the bigotry, blame, and ostracism that afflicted those stricken with the disease circulated in the media. Outside of class, I joined a fledgling AIDS group. I went to meetings attended by the doctors who treated "patient zero," a Montrealer alleged to have started the epidemic. They tried to reassure a nervous public that the epidemic could be brought under control.

Within a few years, friends started to report being sick; some died. I went to medical school. During my hospital rotations, I was assigned the AIDS patients. No one else wanted to look after them. As a medical resident in 1990, I remember one of my professors pulling me aside, asking me why I was so interested in a "dirty" disease. When I started to practice in 1992 in the Montreal General Hospital's AIDS clinic, an average of two patients died every week. In those years I often cycled to the homes of patients who were too sick to come to the hospital or just didn't want to. Several times I was called to pronounce them dead. I cared for an old friend who had returned to Montreal to die. He was joined there by his family and his former partner, Jeff. Jeff asked me whether I would help him organize community groups around HIV in Africa. It was a new approach, he explained. Governments and the big international agencies were unwilling or even unable to do the kind of grassroots organizing necessary to stem the tide. Would I be willing to give some time to work in Africa?

At the clinic in Montreal, African patients had started to appear. There was hardly any discussion of the epidemic coursing through Africa at the time. In Canada, we only had a handful of drugs—AZT, ddI—and they hardly made a dent in the disease's relentless progression. So I couldn't be of much use as a doctor and didn't feel I could be of much use as a community organizer either, I told Jeff. "But you're a physician," he answered, "and people will listen to you." The prejudice and injustice I witnessed with the arrival of AIDS in Montreal had convinced me to go to medical school. The indifference to the AIDS epidemic in Africa—even among those who were committed AIDS activists in the United States and Canada—spurred me to accept Jeff's invitation. I first traveled to Ouagadougou, the capital of Burkina Faso, one of the poorest countries in Africa, in 1994, and then to Abidjan in Côte-d'Ivoire. In these cities I met Abdoulaye, a young community organizer, Dominique, and many others who were trying to respond to this deadly epidemic. This book will follow Abdoulaye, Dominique, and others who struggled with HIV personally and politically during those early years, when an international response began to focus on people living with HIV.

I continued to work part-time at the AIDS clinic in Montreal. During this period, HIV treatment underwent a revolution. Gone were the days of single courses of AZT or ddI. We conducted clinical trials with new drugs. I remember the first clinical trial in 1994 that used one of the new drugs—saquinavir—in combination with two of the older drugs we used to prescribe singly. The results were stunning. In our hospital, patients stopped dying. Some patients were literally resurrected from their deathbeds by the new drugs. I wondered how these miraculous new treatments could get to Africa. But in the AIDS conferences I attended, this was not discussed. The drugs were too expensive. In Africa, it would have to be prevention and perhaps palliative care.

The next time I saw Dominique was a chance encounter in 1996, outside the arrivals area of the Vancouver airport. He had just flown in from Abidjan. The French embassy there had given him a plane ticket to come to the International AIDS conference. He had arrived without any idea of where he was going. At the conference, researchers presented evidence that the new anti-HIV drug cocktails effectively stopped the virus in its tracks and speculated that the drugs might eventually cure AIDS. AIDS activists denounced the news as the false hype of a cynical drug industry and poured fake blood on scientists. When I ran into Dominique that time, his eyes were jaundiced, and he had no place to stay. I debated whether to check him into a hospital or into the university hostel reserved for "developing country delegates" to the conference. Dominique assured me he was fine, and we managed to find a dormitory for him on the university campus.

Dominique died later that year, after he returned to Abidjan. Like other African AIDS activists, he had refused the new treatments, even though his international contacts would have made it possible for him to get the drugs. He told me he would not take the treatments as long as their prohibitive cost put them out of reach of others like him. At the time of his death, it seemed that no Africans—other than the wealthy few—would ever have access to the prohibitively expensive drugs.

Over the next two years, four Ivoirian friends signaled to me they were HIV positive. Marie-Hélène had been sick for a while, and although we never talked openly about her diagnosis, it was understood between us. Ange-Daniel, who was well known for his bisexual promiscuity—his friends often teased him about his frequent visits to the women who sell antibiotics for venereal diseases on the street—confided that he had found out after getting tested at the city's anonymous testing clinic. Solange found out after a bout of illness. It wasn't until the fourth time, when Kouamé told me that he had been tested and was positive, that it dawned on me that they had gotten tested because they knew me. With a Canadian physician as a friend, it had seemed safe to find out.

maybe have options? — Don't want to know if don't have options

Solange went on to join a group of women with HIV. I managed to get medicines to her through a colleague. They kept her healthy, and eventually she managed to cobble together a steady supply so that I didn't have to worry so much about the day my supplies—donated by patients who didn't use up their prescriptions—might run out. The last time I saw her was at an AIDS conference in Barcelona, six years after Dominique died. At the conference's closing ceremony, before Nelson Mandela spoke, a large group of South Africans sang freedom hymns and Solange, who was sitting beside me, wept.

AIDS as kind of oppress"

Telling the Story

This book examines a pivotal moment in the global AIDS epidemic: the period between 1994 and 2000. It does so from the perspective of both local and international efforts to organize communities with HIV in French-speaking West Africa. This period begins with the discovery of effective antiretroviral treatments for HIV in 1994 and ends with the reversal of the international policy consensus that HIV drugs should not be used in Africa because of cost and logistical challenges. Millions lived and died with AIDS during this period, even though treatment existed that could have saved lives. I was driven to write this book to explore and expose the obscene inequality and insidious logic that values lives differently. This was the logic that said that HIV drugs were too expensive for Africans but not for Canadians. It was a logic that began to break down in 2000, thanks to the efforts of a global activist movement.

The Republic of Therapy examines how, in the context of attempts to respond to the epidemic of West Africa, the promise of treatment took hold. It is an ethnography of responses to the epidemic, both local and international; an ethnography of lives lost and lives saved.[2] It also presents a select history of events and people that informed these responses.

As will become clear, this ethnography is as much based on my personal involvement as an activist and physician as on "traditional" fieldwork. As a community organizer with HIV groups in French-speaking West Africa, I wrote grants, trained community workers, and participated in workshops and the everyday life of the groups that I describe throughout the book. I was also recruited to work as a consultant to international organizations involved in responding to HIV in developing countries between 1994 and 2000. I attended meetings, drafted policies, and designed programs; I also led strategic planning exercises and participated in "technical assistance missions" abroad. This gave me valuable insights into the workings of this "industry."

Being an HIV doctor had advantages and drawbacks that are also an important background to the story. While my medical credentials gave me credibility and access, they also influenced my relationships with people, particularly those who were aware they were HIV positive. This was a time when knowing someone like me was their only chance of getting treatment. I became increasingly involved in mobilizing resources and political support for greater access to antiretroviral drugs, even while I cobbled together drug supplies for those I knew needed them. Most doctors need some kind of medical infrastructure to care for people, and this was not available in the kind of work I was doing in West Africa in the mid-1990s. It was not until 1998 that I was able find a clinic in Abidjan that at the time was one of only a few in Africa using antiretroviral drugs, and I began to work there as a volunteer physician.

After clinic hours, I explored Abidjan's urban subcultures, meeting and interviewing members of the self-help groups, psychotherapy circles, and healing cults that populate the city and provided a glimpse into its vibrant therapeutic economy.[3] Everyday life in this city, where social relations easily transport the curious visitor across social worlds, worlds where lasting friendships are made, offered ethnographic insights and illuminates the material presented throughout the book. The archives of medical and social science research institutions in Abidjan were also a treasure-trove of otherwise inaccessible studies.[4] I began to see how Ivoirian history, Abidjan's HIV epidemic, and the responses to it fit together.

The Paradox

As I worked to provide treatment for AIDS in Africa, unintended and sometimes perverse consequences of HIV treatment efforts began to emerge. I was gnawed by the awareness that while these efforts saved lives, they did so in ways that were selective. Not all lives had the same value. I observed how attempts by international and local organizations seeking to respond to the epidemic on humanitarian grounds unwittingly sorted those who should live from those who could go without treatment. This paradox is what I call *triage*. The cultural and political logic of triage persisted in attempts to design, fund, and implement mass treatment programs in the developing world after 2000, and it is visible to this day. The global endeavor to save lives continues to separate those it may most easily rescue—and count—from the rest.

Global health inequalities mean that illness and death stalk the lives of the world's poor. HIV is only the latest in a litany of preventable and treatable diseases that shorten the lives of billions. Tuberculosis and malaria have recently received attention, but diarrheal diseases of children, childbirth, diabetes, and lung and heart conditions are also common and deadly afflictions in developing countries. Working in Africa, every day I observed firsthand the toll these preventable conditions took. Regardless, it seemed that the battle against AIDS was all that mattered. I began to ask myself what forms of politics might emerge in a world where sometimes the only way to survive is by having a fatal illness. It is a politics where the power to save lives is as important as the power to inflict bodily harm or kill. My personal experience and research into the social and political history of Côte-d'Ivoire have led me to conclude that the HIV epidemic and the struggle over access to treatment have heralded a novel form of political power: what I call *therapeutic sovereignty*.

This term is inspired by Mariella Pandolfi's use of the term "mobile sovereignty" (Pandolfi 2000) to describe the humanitarian apparatus that migrated from Kosovo to Albania in the wake of the Balkan wars (see Pandolfi 2006, 2008). There are many ways to define sovereignty, but to me there are none more concise than that of the currently influential German political philosopher Carl Schmitt. Schmitt's revival has as much to do with the fact that his association with the Nazi regime made his ideas unpalatable to all but those on the political right, as with the exceptional political responses in Canada, the United Kingdom, and the United States to the attacks in New York City on 11 September 2001.[5] Schmitt (2005, 5) famously wrote "sovereign is he who decides upon the exception." AIDS has been defined as an exceptional occurrence, worthy of exceptional responses. The informal and formal procedures, protocols, and policies that decide who should live that have played out in the AIDS epidemic in Africa are not technical, medical, or humanitarian issues. Rather, they are mechanisms that decide exceptions in matters of life and death. In the sense of Schmitt, they constitute an exercise of sovereignty. They point to how and by whom power over life is exercised today in the context of international emergencies like the AIDS epidemic.

The Republic of Therapy shows how triage came about as international organizations responded to grim epidemiological figures in Burkina Faso and Côte-d'Ivoire. These international organizations attempted to foster solidarity and self-help by organizing communities with HIV. As local activists such as Abdoulaye and Dominique tried to translate international efforts into pragmatic forms of solidarity, moral economies were made and unmade. New practices to incite people to get tested and talk about living with HIV collided with harsh realities. Those who came out and testified about living with HIV still faced poverty and an apparently untreatable, fatal illness. Nonetheless, once mastered, these new practices of disclosure proved powerful. When effective treatments were discovered in the mid-1990s, political and economic circumstances dictated that they would be unavailable in Africa. Nevertheless, drugs did trickle in, and having a good story about being HIV positive could grant access to them. Although an embryonic, therapeutic citizenship crystallized, solidarities unraveled in the face of processes that triaged who would have access to treatment.

Viewed in historical context, triage echoes earlier, colonial practices deployed in a struggle over sovereignty. Colonial powers sliced and diced the colonial population according to an imposed logic that valued some over others. Here, too, tactical responses bred forms of citizenship that would, later on, coalesce in the realization of national sovereignty with independence from France. However, that sovereignty would be compromised by the economic crisis that followed the Oil Shock of the 1970s and ushered in a global neoliberal era. In Côte-d'Ivoire, the economic miracle unraveled, and the dream of national sovereignty appeared increasingly elusive; new economic and social cleavages fissured everyday life. As access to education was cut off, mastering new skills and tactics on the street was the only way to assure survival. Self-fashioning could be powerful, but it was about survival, not belonging. When new practices of self-help and empowerment arrived in the time of AIDS, they too were used to survive. From colonial times to the era of internationally mandated "structural adjustment," postcolonial countries such as Burkina Faso and Côte-d'Ivoire have been locked in a long war over sovereignty that has made everyday life a battleground. In this context, well-meaning efforts to heal may unleash unsuspected forces.

The first four chapters of *The Republic of Therapy* chronicle the emergence of efforts to organize communities with HIV in West Africa. They also offer an ethnographic and historical perspective on the early years of the rise of the historically unprecedented and massive global intervention into health in the developing world.[6] Chapter 1 begins by showing how embryonic forms of solidarity between people with HIV sutured a "moral economy" that valued contributions to collective survival. However, when international efforts to foster self-help and empowerment for people with HIV introduced new social practices and material resources, they unintentionally disrupted this moral economy. Driven by the need to show results, international organizations privileged testimonials and "body counts" of people living with HIV as evidence of their programs' effectiveness. They began to link funding to evidence that results were being achieved. A strange market for testimonials emerged. But by 1996, the "moral economy" that bound together these early efforts to organize communities with HIV began to unravel.

All across the continent, billboards urged Africans to "get tested" and, in more intimate settings, those who were diagnosed with HIV were being trained—and paid—to give testimonials about their seropositivity. Chapter 2 explores in further detail the attempt to stimulate the production of HIV testimonials and the practice of HIV disclosure through the use of what Nancy Hunt (1997) termed "confessional technologies." These technologies did more than train people to produce narratives of illness. They equipped individuals to talk about themselves and to get others to talk about themselves. The self was made available as a *substrate* that could be examined, prodded, discussed, and worked upon. These incitements to disclose shaped social relations around those who mastered the arts of asking, telling, and listening. They also conjured the "self" into a powerful, life-giving force. In his historico-philosophical analysis of the spiritual exercises of ancient Greece and Rome and the early Christian Church, the French philosopher Michel Foucault showed how forms of discipline, examination of conscience, and bodily practice were used by individuals to fashion themselves in accordance with prevailing moral codes. He called them "technologies of the self" to show how these practices were applied to the raw material, or substrate, of soul and body, and in so doing shaped the way people came to experience and understand themselves as citizens, adepts, or believers. Confessional technologies are an exemplar of technologies of the self.

Chapter 3 asks whether these forms of self-fashioning were really new. Efforts to organize communities with HIV through confessional practice are contrasted with other communities of testimonial practice and forms of association in Côte-d'Ivoire's past and present. Colonial prophetic movements are a striking historical example of how old ways of life could be dissolved in the wake of powerful testimonials borne by charismatic individuals, subsequently allowing new forms of social relations and religious solidarities to emerge. In the colonial period, voluntary associations became social laboratories that allowed experimentation with new forms of self-expression and eventually allowed new forms of charismatic practice to emerge. In late-twentieth-century Côte-d'Ivoire, prophecy was both charismatic and routine. I explore how one church, the Spiritual Ministry of the Soldiers of God, linked the spiritual and the bureaucratic through individualized testimonial practices that I refer to as an "administration of prophecies." In contrast with the growing competitiveness and schism in HIV groups, when the solidarity of shared disclosure began to dissolve as competition for resources intensified, the Soldiers of God used prophecy to produce a pragmatic solidarity that bound people together within the church. While self-fashioning existed from colonial times, the technologies deployed in the war on AIDS mobilized a newly powerful form of selfhood.

This can be seen in Chapter 4, which follows how confessional technologies furnished the tools for some of those living with HIV to become proficient advocates. These patient-activists were among the first to benefit from the life-saving antiretroviral (ARV) drugs that began to trickle into Africa in the late 1990s, smuggled in by fellow activists from the North. This experience shaped what I have called a "therapeutic citizenship," as people living with HIV developed a powerful sense of rights and responsibilities inherent to their medical predicament. As the trickle of drugs increased to a stream, decisions had to be made about which members in these early community groups should benefit. Confessional technologies trained people to talk about themselves, and talking about yourself came to be about staying alive.

The first formal treatment programs finally arrived, along with explicit criteria as to who should be treated; however, behind these conditions were unexamined assumptions about which patients would be most "adherent" to the drugs and therefore most likely to benefit from their therapeutic effect. Clinical trials, pilot programs, and treatment activism operated under different criteria of who should be privileged for treatment. Life itself was subjected to different calculations of value. These processes of selection further fissured the fragile moral economy of HIV groups, as a logic of solidarity gave way to one of triage.

"Triage" is a medical term used to describe procedures for prioritizing those who must receive medical care immediately over those who may wait. While triage was initially developed on the battlefield to sort out soldiers who could be treated and return to combat from those who could not, it is an everyday facet of medical practice in emergency rooms, where nurses prioritize patients for care based on the severity of their condition. In its original conception, triage is a calculation that seeks to optimize the use of scarce resources to preserve combat-ready manpower rather than to save lives. In its everyday, civilian use, triage seeks to allocate medical care to those who need it most urgently in order to save lives, so that a patient with a potentially fatal heart attack, for instance, would not be kept waiting while a broken arm is set. In medicine, then, triage can be deployed to different ends, based on criteria that value life differently.[7] In the case of early efforts to organize communities with HIV, triage occurred when separate and unrelated social practices gradually intertwined. Technical and bureaucratic procedures for singling out people for help, narrative practices of disclosure (and of "telling" the truth about the self), and self-transformation became linked in the struggle to gain access to life-saving treatment. Triage in the time of AIDS thus brought together three types of practices (differentiation, truth telling, and self-transformation) in ways that, wittingly or not, determined who should live and who might die.

Differentiation, Zero-Sum Economics, and Accusation in Côte-d'Ivoire

Did these forms of triage emerge because of local quirks or internationally imposed constraints? Or was it a bit of both? What might be the social implications of triage? The second part of this book attempts to answer these questions. It explores the historical trajectory in Côte d'Ivoire that led practices of differentiation, survival tactics in a time of scarcity, and "telling the truth" about oneself to converge in the time of AIDS. A global dynamic of expropriation has held Côte d'Ivoire firmly in its grasp since colonial conquest. Earlier inequalities traced social fault-lines between Africans and Europeans, city-dwellers and peasants, and ethnic groups "made up" by colonial authorities. These social fault-lines were prone to fissure as newer economic stresses came along. Violence and forms of truth telling proliferated at these sites of cleavage. New forms of economic, social, and political exclusion occurred, most visibly in exceptional times, where matters of life and death were at stake: during the wars of colonial conquest, the epidemics that threatened the young colony, and the revolts and uprisings that have since punctuated the history of Côte-d'Ivoire. Triage in the time of AIDS is but the most recent facet of this long history.

Chapter 5 elaborates on the concept of biopower to trace the long historical arc that connects colonial and postcolonial struggles over sovereignty to contemporary forms of triage in the time of AIDS. In the colonial period, France's sovereignty over Côte-d'Ivoire faced two threats: epidemics and violent resistance on the part of those colonized. Dividing practices provided a unified approach to managing both. The violence of colonial conquest persisted in a more subtle form as colonial authorities segregated Africans from settlers in the name of health. Crude policies of segregation then gave way to more finely grained economic and governmental practices that drew on ethnographic knowledge to sort Africans into distinct groups. Even after independence, government policies shaped urban life and citizenship by producing new forms of division. Despite the flawed knowledge on which these practices were based, they nonetheless produced new social relations and, in the process, "made up" new kinds of people who spoke out and even resisted these attempts to impose a social order. Here we can see a historical parallel with contemporary efforts to respond to HIV. With historical hindsight, it is now possible to see how voluntary and ethnic forms of association, and even prophetic "truth telling" that framed the ethical dilemmas of colonial subjects, later coalesced into larger political formations that, at the time, would have been unimaginable: African nationalism, the postcolonial state and its politics, urban cultures and ways of life. As we look deeper into the history, it becomes clear that what is at stake in triage is none other than sovereignty: who gets to exert power over life.

Chapter 6 explores how in Côte-d'Ivoire a period of "miraculous" economic growth through the 1960s crashed abruptly in the late 1970s, cleaving society along the stark economic contrasts that resulted. The state increasingly appeared unable to deliver on the promises of modernity. National sovereignty eroded as international agencies intervened in the economy. The crisis ushered in a long downward spiral. A parallel "shadow" economy proliferated among the ruins of what had been a vibrant "modern" economy. The unraveling economy bred a zero-sum cultural logic, whereby the acquisition of wealth could only occur at the expense of the poor. Survival became a matter of social relations, ingenuity, discipline, and quick-wittedness, rather than formal qualification. Schooling was replaced by self-fashioning, and life in the city was a training ground for "street warriors." A depleted state and an increasing sense that national sovereignty was of little practical value left few options but to resort to technologies of the self. Foreshadowing how this would play out in the fight against AIDS, these technologies empowered only a few and created new social divisions.

Narrative practices, particularly the incitement to tell the "truth" about one's self, became mechanisms for sorting people and a basis for rationing access to treatment in the time of AIDS. Confessional technologies were used to help people overcome so-called cultural barriers to disclosure, such as prudishness around sexual matters or "stigma" around HIV. However, disclosures about intimate matters were already powerfully linked to desire, money, and power within a broader economy of secrecy. Chapter 7 begins by exploring how in Abidjan, the socioeconomic fissures opened up by the crisis even led to what was called a "war of the sexes," as men lost jobs and economic ground to women. As social and economic inequalities widened, the city's reputation for sexual liberalism linked sexuality and economy in myriad ways. In the subterranean world of rumor and gossip, economic and sexual desires blended even as economic anxieties generated widespread suspicions of moral decay in the last years of the twentieth century. Corruption and forbidden sexualities could be known only by those who were directly engaged, binding them in an economy of secrecy. This final chapter explores how, as economic conditions worsened and evidence of political dysfunction became endemic, the moral imagination linked corruption and forbidden sex. In this toxic atmosphere, disrupting this economy of secrecy could be perilous, unleashing suspicion and even unsuspected forces. "Confession" in this context was also accusation. As Côte-d'Ivoire's First Republic unraveled, earlier cleavages channeled the violence that exploded.

The Exception

The contemporary "politics" of AIDS are not those of colonial times, but they nonetheless demonstrate parallels in the way that foreign powers continue to intervene in Africa—no longer to kill and conquer but to ensure that certain populations (such as those living with HIV) may live. Interventions have multiplied with the recognition that the epidemic is no less than a humanitarian emergency, requiring exceptional measures so that lives may be saved. The term "AIDS exceptionalism" is often used to stress that the response to the epidemic must, and does, differ from other public health interventions. As a humanitarian emergency, AIDS now defines exception in epidemiological terms. But it has become an issue that may, in fragmented and partial ways, suspend national sovereignty. The emergency has mobilized a loose assemblage of transnational institutions and local groups that, in the exceptional case of AIDS, exercise powers that effectively decide who lives and who dies. AIDS relief efforts are thus political in the strongest sense, projecting the power of life or death, and doing so through an apparatus that has linked truth telling to a vast epidemiological machinery for sorting out people. What are the political formations that may result from this mobile and partial therapeutic sovereignty? May not a kind of "republic of therapy" emerge from its shadow?

TESTIMONIALS THAT BIND

. . . .

Organizing Communities with HIV

In 1990, a young man named Abdoulaye traveled from Abidjan to Ouagadougou, six hundred kilometers to the north in Burkina Faso, where he went on to found a youth group, Jeunes sans frontières (Youth without Borders). He had just turned twenty-seven when I first met him in 1995. I begin with Abdoulaye's story because it reveals the complexity of organizing communities living with HIV in West Africa. There, the impact of international efforts to organize communities with HIV intersected in unpredictable ways with everyday attempts to grapple with matters of life and death. Western assumptions that solidarity and self-help could result from a shared biomedical condition were lost in translation. Abdoulaye's story shows how this happened.

Shy and soft-spoken, with a tendency to speak quietly while using a self-effacing first person plural, for those around him, Abdoulaye was different from others his age. His uncles treated him almost as an equal, according him more respect than those in his age-class and more even than his older brother. That this never caused any tension was evidence of Abdoulaye's skill at balancing the needs of family hierarchy with his own aspirations. Neither he nor his cousins and friends attributed this to his personality—for them, it came from his being born south of the border in Abidjan and being wise in the ways of fast life in the big city. Work motivated Abdoulaye's parents to move to Abidjan in the 1960s, when the Ivoirian economic "miracle" was still in full swing, fuelled by favorable global market prices for the country's primary exports of cocoa and coffee. Abdoulaye's parents found work in the booming economy: his mother in a plastics factory and his father at the port, the major clearinghouse along the coast for the interior and the landlocked countries of Mali, Burkina Faso, and Niger to the north. In their trek south, Abdoulaye's parents had followed a well-worn path — the migration route between Burkina Faso and Côte-d'Ivoire dates from the earliest colonial times.[1]

Abdoulaye grew up in the Abidjan township of Anoumabo, formerly an Ébrié village on the lagoon, which had long ago been swallowed up by the sprawl of the city and had become home to many Burkinabè. His older brother stayed, their father having found him a job at the port, but Abdoulaye wanted to continue his schooling. Abdoulaye's family could not afford to keep him in school in Côte-d'Ivoire, where school fees were higher, and foreigners were not eligible for the few scholarships available.[2] So, after he finished his secondary school in Abidjan, Abdoulaye returned to Ouagadougou to go to university in 1990. Once there, he moved into the ancestral home: a cement house around a courtyard, inhabited by his father's three brothers, each with three wives, and each with "five or six" children. The family got by reasonably comfortably; although illiterate, the uncles were successful merchants, and the wives managed small businesses out of the home. They sold charcoal, made fried doughnuts to sell to passers-by, and used the capital they accumulated to buy bags of rice and millet that they resold in smaller parcels.

Abdoulaye spent a year at the university in Ouagadougou, but the transition was difficult. Ouagadougou was not like Abidjan, and he couldn't shake the feeling that he didn't quite belong. Perhaps this was why Abdoulaye became interested in the way others his age lived in Ouagadougou and the problems they faced. Maybe his desire to be involved was a way to reconcile his feelings of being different. With his analytic mind and good writing skills, Abdoulaye quickly learned that he didn't need to finish university to make a niche for himself. He experimented with writing project proposals for development agencies, and some of them were funded. Ouagadougou had become a center for these agencies for several reasons; droughts had devastated the countryside, and Burkina had a reputation for being receptive to development agencies. After the droughts of the 1970s had thankfully passed, the development agencies stayed to focus on other problems, including family planning. Abdoulaye came along when family planning had already been embraced as the solution to poverty, and attention was beginning to turn to the importance of educating young girls about contraception. These interventions were the forerunners of subsequent AIDS-education campaigns.

Organizations such as Abdoulaye's did not work in a vacuum; it was their embeddedness in local social relations and networks of obligation and reciprocity that gave them their credibility and the local knowledge that was so valuable to international agencies. A large part of their work as subcontractors to large development agencies was to translate these social policies into locally meaningful knowledge and practice. Jeunes sans frontières invested family-planning money in creating jobs for local youth as peer-educators or outreach workers. In exchange for the labor that kept projects going, Abdoulaye paid his youthful charges a decent wage. Their enthusiasm impressed the organization's funders. Shrewdly, the organization used these investments to develop a multivalent infrastructure—neighborhood kiosks, a central office, scooters—onto which other money-generating projects could be piggybacked.

Abdoulaye and I often met at the Jeunes sans frontières office, which served both as a headquarters and a social center. Young men and women, presumably from the group's various "antennae" (as Abdoulaye liked to call them) in the city, would drop by on errands or to request advice, more often than not lingering, the women chatting outside or the young men draping themselves over the three rickety chairs grouped around a table. Gradually I would learn that many of these young people, the inner circle of the organization, were related to Abdoulaye as cousins, brothers, or sisters. Abdoulaye relied on family members, not so much as a result of crude patronage, but because the presence of kinship ties meant that these individuals could be trusted. In a setting of dire poverty and social precariousness, it was difficult to trust people one did not know and who were not tied by the obligations kinship afforded. Others who joined the organization and established a reputation for reliability and "seriousness" became *like* family. Some even moved into Abdoulaye's family's compound.

As in many parts of the world, in Ouagadougou people live in extended families, sharing a series of rooms organized around a central courtyard where meals are cooked. Kinship was an idiom for describing social relatedness, not so much in defining one's identity as in identifying to whom one may turn in a time of need.[4] Abdoulaye was stitching together a network of social relations where kinship relations and obligations furnished the idiom through which accountability and hierarchy could be expressed and relation-

adapter

ships valued. Jeunes sans frontières' success was less a product of good management practice than of Abdoulaye's skill at suturing this hybrid network of friends, family, and sympathizers to the abstract programs of international agencies. He capitalized on his kinship-ordered social relations to build a community organization; this was his "charisma." As will become clear over the next three chapters in this book, however, the idiom of kinship hides more than it reveals in this study of HIV groups.

New Opportunities with AIDS

By 1995 AIDS had become of major concern for development agencies. The epidemiological statistics were worrisome—the epidemic was exploding to the south, particularly in Abidjan, and the figures from Burkina seemed to indicate that the epidemic was also progressing there. It was widely believed that HIV traveled through the migratory system from Abidjan, thought to be the epicenter of the epidemic in West Africa,[5] to Burkina Faso. Abdoulaye and his parents were part of the estimated three million Burkinabè who divided their lives between Burkina Faso and Côte-d'Ivoire (Cordell, Gregory, and Piché 1996). Some moved to Abidjan for work and then stayed, or else returned to Burkina for school. The more usual pattern was for young men to leave the agriculturally desolate areas of northern Burkina Faso to labor on the plantations or in the city (as servants, gardeners, car attendants, or working in any of the myriad jobs in the big city's informal economy) and then to return to the village to marry once they saved up enough money. It is this pattern that was believed to have extended the reach of the epidemic from the metropolis of Abidjan as far as the isolated villages on the edge of the Sahara, thousands of kilometers to the north.

mobility

When I first met him in 1995, Abdoulaye had already developed an impressive list of credentials. Several projects he had put together had been funded and successfully carried out. The introductions he was writing to his project proposals were ethnographic treatises in their own right, effortlessly citing demographic statistics alongside observations about the sexual lives of urban youth and incisive analyses about the cultural barriers to addressing issues of sexuality. Development agencies had been quick to respond, and Jeunes sans frontières had already been carrying out family planning education campaigns for two years. As a result, the organization had chapters in over a dozen neighborhoods. This had given Abdoulaye the opportunity to embellish his project proposals with the wealth of information he had gathered through his involvement in these campaigns.

For the family planning campaigns, Abdoulaye recruited articulate young people and trained them as peer-educators: youth that educate other youth about the importance of contraception. This allowed him to pay them modest fees from the contracts, and with the small overheads he earned from these, he was able to rent a modest office on a busy road not far from his house. When AIDS appeared on the agenda of the development agencies in 1994, the major emphasis was not on medical treatment—after all, even though anti-HIV drugs (antiretrovirals, or ARVs) had existed since the discovery of AZT in 1989, the lifesaving combination ARV "cocktails" had only been reported that year, and the drugs were prohibitively expensive, costing thousands of dollars a month. In Africa, then, the emphasis was on preventing HIV by raising awareness and encouraging condom use—the family planning strategy with which Abdoulaye and the group were most familiar.

Jeunes sans frontières' initial experience with HIV activities was during the World AIDS Day events, on 1 December, starting in 1993. Abdoulaye told me these were "great fun." The National AIDS Program could be counted on to hand out small grants to do "awareness-raising" during the government-organized AIDS parade, and the colorful NGO stands lent a festive air to the proceedings. There would be shows, giveaways of T-shirts and rubbers, and the obligatory displays of putting condoms onto wooden penises.

An Epidemic of Visibility

Given his experience with World AIDS Day and family-planning campaigns, Abdoulaye found it easy to retool his organization to respond to the development agencies' new priority. He told me he was glad he could stay in the business of educating people about sexuality; it was interesting, as was the research it entailed. He could investigate intriguing questions: why young girls would sleep with older men even if they had boyfriends (he found out it was to pay for school fees and clothes); why most of the tailors in Ouagadougou were Ghanaian (access to cheaper hair clippers in Ghana gave them a competitive advantage and they had cornered the market before anyone else). He could then use the answers to improve on subsequent project proposals.

The Jeunes sans frontières office was equipped with a typewriter and a shelf stacked with glossy family-planning brochures and decorated with three

AIDS posters: One from Uganda showed a photo of a gaunt man with his two children on a bench and below, in English, "I had lost hope. You counseled me. TASO — The AIDS Support Organisation." Another poster, this one from Côte-d'Ivoire, featured a dying man on a cot in a hospital, his eyes blanked out with a black rectangle: "I have AIDS. Don't abandon me. National AIDS Control Programme." The third, from America, had an incongruously colorful picture of the virus and its genetic components. Although lit by a naked light bulb, the office still appeared dark, with green walls and a ceiling fan that always seemed ineffective against both the heat and the dust on the brochures. The images on these posters were still a distant reality for Abdoulaye. He knew the figures for Burkina (at the time 10 percent of the population was estimated to have been contaminated by HIV; that figure is now recognized to have been an overestimation[6]), but he had never met anyone who was HIV positive. Nonetheless, he believed the problem was there. He knew most youth didn't use condoms, and given the statistics, it was evident that the virus was spreading. In this, Abdoulaye had come to the same conclusion as the development agencies. This was why, by late 1995, international agencies were getting concerned about the HIV epidemic. Despite the proliferation of condom promotion campaigns, they had the nagging sensation that no one was taking the problem seriously enough. "It's all just theater," one development official told me, adding "IEC [Information-Education-Communication, as such condom promotion campaigns were called] activities won't lead to sustainable behavior change." For the international agencies, the proof was that no one seemed to talk about AIDS "unless they're paid to." There were no press articles or other manifestations of "genuine concern." The term "silent epidemic" was used interchangeably with "invisible epidemic" to describe the situation, which was inevitably contrasted with the alarming figures drawn from seroprevalence studies.[7]

Both officially and off the record, the lack of "visibility" of the epidemic was decried as a major "barrier" to combating the disease and evidence of "denial." These claims would have been bolstered by a visit to the local hospital; there, the epidemic was clearly visible to the clinically trained eye. Physicians who practiced in Burkina's public health system privately acknowledged seeing clinical cases of AIDS starting in the late 1980s, but were unable to confirm their suspicions because of the lack of tests and the impression that diagnosing HIV infections was not really considered important at the time.

This clinical visibility didn't translate into the kind of visibility the development agencies wanted. In the early years, HIV-testing kits were rarely available, and even if they were, patients were still not told of their diagnosis. Winston, a nurse in one of the main medical wards, once showed me a stack of patients' charts in the small room where he slept on night shifts. Patients with positive tests results had the result clearly indicated, with the hospital's diagnostic code for HIV infection ("1762") on their chart; about three-quarters of the patients in this ward had the number inked in red on their charts. However, only a handful had the letter "A" (for "announced") beside it, meaning that they had been told. Winston gave a simple reason for not informing the patients: "Patients aren't told because it would only discourage them." In his experience, patients who were told went on to die very quickly. His ward was divided into two sections—one for more acute cases and one for more chronic cases. Patients with HIV were triaged to the chronic section. But, Winston explained, "once an HIV patient gets transferred to the chronic section, he realizes that he has HIV even if he hasn't been told, and he rarely lasts more than a few days."

Abdoulaye, meanwhile, was encouraged that two of his projects, which had been funded by a European embassy and a British organization, were underway and seemed to be working, at least in terms of the goals he had set for them. Young women were buying and reselling condoms he was purchasing from an American social marketing program,[8] as were the young Ghanaian barbers whom he supplied with condoms and had persuaded to use disposable razors.

A Market for Testimonials

In Côte-d'Ivoire, to the south of Burkina Faso, the HIV epidemic was the focus of much greater attention than in Burkina Faso, where Abdoulaye worked. In the bustling Ivoirian metropolis of Abidjan, the economic stakes of an epidemic were higher, and a well-funded research infrastructure had already underlined the seriousness of the epidemic by demonstrating that HIV had become the leading cause of death (De Cock et al. 1989, 1990 and De Cock, Barrere, Lafontaine, Diaby, Gnaore, Pantobe, and Odehouri 1991). As a result of its economic and epidemiological importance, Abidjan had become an important target of international efforts to combat AIDS in the region. In 1994, the same year I first met Abdoulaye, I began to work in the city where he was born and grew up, Abidjan, and I started to piece together the story behind the first public HIV testimonials. Staff of international agencies recalled to me how they had looked on approvingly as three young people stepped forward to "come out" as HIV positive during a meeting organized to discuss the AIDS problem in 1994, with government officials and local groups in attendance. "At last, to have been able to see these courageous young people affirming themselves," sighed one World Bank official, Madame Janvier, when I asked her to recount what happened at the meeting.

It was a moment of vindication for her and others in the "donor community" (as the ensemble of development agencies are often referred to collectively). Their suspicions of government indifference to the AIDS crisis, nurtured by a perceived history of denial by African governments in the 1980s, had hardened after years of trying to pressure the government to act, with little in the way of concrete results. Development workers regularly complained to me that African governments implemented internationally funded programs at a snail's pace, held endless seminars, and haggled over details. In many respects this was business as usual: seminars were needed, after all, for agencies to explain their programs and train those who would carry them out (whether government workers or NGOs). These workshops initiated participants into the intricacies of the financial accounting, paperwork, and vocabulary of particular programs. The functionaries who attended the workshops were only too happy to get away from the office for a day and, most importantly, to earn a daily fee, or per diem, for attending the workshop.[9] The standardized language of the development industry measured success in terms of outputs, outcomes, impacts, and indicators, measures of value whose limitations were visible to Madame Janvier and others. The consequences of the epidemic were "dramatic," she said, recounting her travels to hospitals in various parts of the country. The figures were bad enough, but to see the suffering that she saw in those hospitals and to know that barely anything that could have an impact was being done was of great concern to her. Things could not continue "as per usual" when it came to AIDS. The statistics, program indicators, and administrative protocols of the development industry traced the outlines of a *moral economy* in which Madame Janvier and Abdoulaye both found themselves when they sought to confront AIDS.

The notion of a moral economy has gained widespread currency in the social sciences since its introduction by the historian Edward P. Thompson (1971). Thompson coined this term to describe social conflicts that emerged between opposing systems of value in response to the rise of the market economy in seventeenth-century England. In anthropology, while moral economies were initially associated with peasant societies (see Scott 1976), the notion has since taken on a broader significance as it has been used to analyze witchcraft (Austen 1993) and corruption in the African context.[10] I use the term here in the manner of Newell (2006, 180), who in a thoughtful ethnographic study of an Abidjan neighborhood, explains:

> By moral economy, I denote a system in which people often exchange for the purpose of maintaining and accumulating social relations, rather than merely for the purpose of maximizing their profits. Of course, in some more abstract sense, people profit from their social relationships, but the point is that the social relationships take priority, or rather, that the maintenance and accumulation of these relationships is its own kind of profit.

The three young people who first came forward to testify about being HIV positive at that 1994 meeting were Dominique, Jeanne, and Étienne. They went on to form Côte-d'Ivoire's first organization of people living with HIV/AIDS and became the darlings of the development agencies. Funding for AIDS groups became readily available, as well as invitations and plane tickets to meetings abroad. But later, Madame Janvier came to have regrets. She felt that it was all "too much" for them: "They always look exhausted, they're always on airplanes. It's too much for their health." Madame Janvier was not alone in singling out the tendency of the new activists to travel frequently. It was a source of much jealousy on the part of those who joined the new organization, while other aid workers occasionally accused colleagues of "showing off" their "pet" HIV-positive Africans at international conferences in a game of one-upmanship.

By placing a premium on finding "real" Africans with HIV, the international community inadvertently fostered competition over public HIV testimonials. This was particularly evident in West Africa, where people who were living with HIV and were willing to talk about it were slow to come forward. By then, southern and eastern African countries like Uganda, which had more advanced epidemics, had organizations that could speak about "living positively" and "counseling," as well as iconic figures—artists, relatives of politicians—who were openly HIV positive. Perhaps the development agencies that made up the donor community were reacting to the frustrations of the Madame Janviers in their ranks, so that, somehow, during the mid-1990s, producing "real" people with HIV came to be seen as evidence that "something is being done." Officially, testimonies by people living with HIV were seen as evidence that "supportive environments" were being created, including the right context for "effective prevention," which would result in "sustainable behavior change." Members of the donor community regularly emphasized their belief that having openly HIV-positive Africans talk about their situation would be taken far more seriously by their compatriots than merely demonstrating condoms at a World AIDS Day fair booth.

In 1995, Jeanne travelled from Côte-d'Ivoire to Burkina Faso to testify about being HIV positive. Her testimonial was broadcast on Burkinabè television. As I mentioned earlier, in the mid-1990s, Burkina Faso was still relatively isolated from the AIDS awareness campaigns that had already blanketed Abidjan with prevention messages. When Jeanne's testimonial aired, people laughed and said that she didn't have HIV because she looked too healthy. "She's doing it for the money," they said.[11] The disbelief that greeted Jeanne's testimonial was a sign that Madame Janvier's (and her colleagues') assumptions were mistaken. In a setting where one did not disclose intimate and painful matters in public, such testimonials could trigger suspicion rather than solidarity. Jeanne returned to Côte-d'Ivoire after her television appearance, but she left behind a precedent that would entangle Abdoulaye as he sought to placate his organization's donors and translate between shifting notions of solidarity and self-help.

A Brief Genealogy of AIDS Testimonials

Getting people living with HIV to testify publicly about being HIV positive is a strategy with a complex genealogy that extends back across the Atlantic and to the circumstances that led to the inextricable linkage of experience with activism in the 1990s (Mann and Tarantola 1996). At the time, a large proportion of those involved in the growth of the AIDS industry already had personal experience with the illness. As a new epidemic disease that was immediately identified with specific social groups, HIV and discrimination went hand-in-hand, reflecting an age-old dynamic where epidemics are a fertile terrain for exclusionary discourses and practices.[12] Since it tended to affect groups that were already marginalized and subject to discrimination,[13] HIV was a potent stigmatizing force. In response, a powerful activist movement emerged in the West that pioneered community-based prevention and care approaches and advocated for more government attention to the epidemic. This activism helped to reorient public health approaches to the epidemic from a narrow, biomedical focus on diagnosis and control to one of inclusion and empowerment (Seidel 1993). This historically unprecedented response was instrumental in decreasing new HIV infections, particularly in the gay community, where activist efforts had been concentrated, and containing the epidemic in Northern countries. Control of the epidemic in the gay community had been achieved through adapted prevention campaigns; for example, posting explicit advice in bathhouses. AIDS activism played a part in treatment breakthroughs through the forceful lobbying of the pharmaceuticals industry, putting pressure on regulatory authorities to fast-track the licensing of drugs ("to get drugs into bodies"), and mobilizing patients to participate in clinical trials (S. Epstein 1996).

This experience shaped the programs that development organizations designed to address the AIDS epidemic in developing countries. Many Northern AIDS activists were hired to key positions in international organizations and brought with them experiences of community development and patient empowerment. This approach was supported by evidence that the active involvement of the gay community and of people living with HIV had been instrumental in achieving public health results. The ideology of patient empowerment went with earlier struggles that resisted "medicalization." This refers to the increasing impetus, beginning in the 1960s and 1970s, for many aspects of life to be framed in biomedical terms as "diseases" requiring intervention. Increasingly, technological interventions were managed by specialist-experts within a growing health care bureaucracy, adding a dehumanizing aspect to biomedicine.[14] As Europe and North America were swept by a diverse array of countercultural movements with roots in the American civil-rights movement in the late 1960s, a robust resistance to medicalization emerged. For instance, feminists pointed to biomedical control over their bodies, particularly with respect to reproduction, as an intolerable manifestation of patriarchy. This radical political stance gained wide resonance throughout American society at the time. Even women who did not share this political analysis widely experienced the paternalist dimensions of biomedical practice (Lock 1988b).

Therefore, the notions of community development and patient empowerment that AIDS activism advocated emerged from the social environment that existed when the epidemic appeared in the major cities of North America in 1981. Widespread ambivalence about the biomedical establishment informed ideas of patient empowerment and community development. At the time, the gay community's sense of identity was an oppositional one, strengthened by landmark events such as the Stonewall riots and by shared experiences of homophobia. The community was deeply suspicious of biomedicine, particularly in light of the fact that medical practitioners widely viewed homosexuality as a disease.[15] In this setting, solidarity was strong and lent itself readily to the creation of a network of community institutions. When the AIDS epidemic came along, this model of self-organizing in the gay community was reproduced in those organizations that sprang up to offer care and support outside of biomedical institutions that were often hostile toward gay men. These included organizations providing services to people with AIDS (such as New York City's Gay Men's Health Crisis) and treatment activist groups (such as ACT-UP; see Kayal 1993). Facilitated by a similar epidemiological distribution (the epidemic affecting largely gay men in the early years), the Anglo-American model of activism spread quickly to Canada, Northwest Europe, and Australia. It was from this network of organizations and their collective experiences that international agencies recruited personnel and drew lessons for designing and implementing AIDS control programs across the world.

The strategy of getting people with HIV to "come out" and give public testimonials was therefore a logical extension of the experience with the epidemic in North America and Europe. Activist experience with the epidemic in North America led to a consensus within international agencies that people with HIV were the key to fighting the epidemic. The logic was that HIV-positive people would help to overcome the perceived "denial" of Africans by "giving a face" to the epidemic. Making the numbers "real," it was believed, would help make people change their behavior. Who wants to wear a condom simply because of a public health message or a statistical construct? People with HIV and AIDS were believed to be closest to the "realities" of HIV and AIDS, and since they were on the "frontlines" of the epidemic, they were the best positioned to react. This view became official dogma at the Paris World AIDS Summit in November 1994, where the Greater Involvement of People with AIDS (GIPA) initiative was ratified by the countries attending, essentially becoming the official policy of the "donor community."[16] For those in the AIDS industry, GIPA represented an important milestone: the acknowledgment at the highest levels that people living with HIV and AIDS were not victims or objects of policy but should take on a leadership role. It was a victory over discourses of exclusion, representing a watershed in the history of public health. This was a turning point whose precondition was the politicization that had occurred in the 1960s and 70s in the countercultural movements. As personal experience—such as women's experiences of male domination in the clinic or in marriage—became political, personal experience came to define new political struggles.

AIDS testimonials therefore came to be considered a necessary part of efforts to control the epidemic. International agencies actively sought out testimonials and encouraged local authorities to incite people with HIV to come out publicly. International agencies pointed to the presence of testimonials in other countries as evidence that a "culture of denial" around the epidemic was dissipating and that the fight against AIDS was progressing. Such evidence, it should be added, would help keep monetary support for activities aimed at combating the AIDS epidemic flowing.

seeking/ paying for testmnl even using as evd da ol cltrl △

The First Testimonial in Ouagadougou

The year after Abdoulaye's second World AIDS Day, in mid-July 1995, he came across a letter, published in the Ouagadougou newspaper *L'Observateur Paalga*:

> I am a twenty-seven-year-old man, and I live in a neighborhood of the capital. But I will have to leave this neighborhood, where I have lived for ten years, because I am singled out and my neighbors who know me well flee me. The last few months have been hell for me. Even when I feel like having a beer in the bar next door, the customers get up, quickly settle their bills, timidly say good-bye to me and disappear. Others, often, buy me a beer, and when I get up to shake their hands and thank them, they refuse to shake my hand. It's unbearable for me—and I've done nothing wrong. I have neither stolen, or beaten anyone, or raped anyone. My crime is to be seropositive, and AIDS, this disease that frightens so, has terrorized my neighborhood where I lived peacefully until everyone found out. I have lived through desperate moments. At home, when the meal is ready, no one wants to sit to eat with me. Everyone manages to eat before or after me; never at the same time. But my portion of food is always kept for me and is always generous. My mechanic refuses to fix my moped because, according to him, I may have cut myself and if my blood has touched the engine, he could contaminate himself. He told this to his apprentices: "Money, sure, but my life comes first!" What is happening to me is a scandal. Those like me who have contracted this horrible disease need to communicate,

to feel loved and that we are not different from others. We know that we have little time left to live; so we must not give up hope. Why make us suffer even more in our bodies, in our spirit, and in our hearts?[17]

By the time the letter was published, Jeunes sans frontières had multiplied its successes at fundraising. Abdoulaye, with his youthful management team, had opened up a string of AIDS awareness cafés staffed by peer-educators across the city. These kiosks sold Nescafé, soft drinks, and condoms. That these "educators" seemed more interested in catching up on the latest political gossip with customers and selling sandwiches seemed to confirm the development agencies' worries that their prevention campaigns weren't getting very far. But for Abdoulaye this was Jeunes sans frontières' most practical accomplishment so far. The prevention cafés allowed the association to employ some of the young people who had been volunteering in his group—young people who would otherwise have had no source of income. As Abdoulaye pointed out, this made it significantly less likely that they would be tempted to exchange sex for money and put themselves at risk of getting HIV. The cafés also turned a small profit, giving the association a valuable financial cushion in case grants didn't come through or donor funding unexpectedly dried up. This gave them an important measure of independence from donor-driven imperatives.

A few weeks before World AIDS Day of 1996, Abdoulaye told me about reading the letter. He responded to it by writing back to the newspaper that published his letter. Abdoulaye offered the support of Jeunes sans frontières to the author of the letter. The young man who wrote the letter, Issa, came to the organization's office, and Abdoulaye eventually put him to work delivering bottles of soft drinks to the kiosks.

Abdoulaye told me that his response to Issa's letter in the paper was an opportunity to respond to a situation he believed to be "real" but that he hadn't been able to address directly as he hadn't met anyone with HIV until meeting Issa. He pointed out that the HIV seroprevalence figures, which he could recite by heart from writing up project proposals, meant that he knew that people with HIV were "out there." And perhaps he was also curious. Until he met Issa, "all this AIDS business" remained somewhat of an abstraction to him. Issa's story certainly corresponded to what Abdoulaye expected. His account of rejection and solitude echoed the posters on the walls of the office. Abdoulaye was used to dealing with young people in difficult situations: no income, living with families that couldn't afford to feed them. Abdoulaye felt Issa needed "special" help right away because of his "situation." But how to offer it without singling Issa out? "Issa needs to talk, and one of these days he'll need medicines he won't be able to afford, even with the small income we can give him," Abdoulaye told me. Abdoulaye was faced with a dilemma: Issa's apparent need to talk about his experience of being HIV positive could not be addressed by adopting Issa into the extended family of Jeunes sans frontières.

Abdoulaye never told anyone about Issa's HIV positivity until much later. Abdoulaye confided to me about Issa because I was an "outsider," someone who could be expected not to tell. Abdoulaye once told me that "the African feels that he can trust the White man . . . because they're not like us, they don't go around telling everyone everyone's secrets." Whiteness meant being outside the network of rumor and gossip that could threaten a reputation and a livelihood.[18] As a result, he introduced me to Issa because he felt that Issa would be able to "open up" to me about his HIV positivity. But Issa did not confide more to me than he had to Abdoulaye. For him, even though we were both trustworthy, and I could offer medical reassurance, Abdoulaye had the position of a "senior brother" (even though, in fact, Abdoulaye was younger than Issa) because he had taken on the burden of Issa's secret and would "look after" him.

But, that November of 1996, Issa's trust in his new senior brother took on added ramifications. Even before Issa's arrival, Abdoulaye had for some time been dropping hints in his dealings with his organization's funders that there were people with HIV among the ranks of Jeunes sans frontières. He told me he knew that this disclosure would give him additional legitimacy with the development agencies; and besides, given the seroprevalence rates, it had to be the case, even if he didn't know anyone who had been officially diagnosed in the group. No doubt as a result of Abdoulaye's strategic hints, in the weeks leading up to World AIDS Day on 1 December, he was approached by an influential member of the National AIDS Committee, which was desperately looking for someone to testify publicly on television on World AIDS Day. Since he knew some HIV-positive youth, would he be able to approach them so that they could do this, "face uncovered"? Abdoulaye saw a unique opportunity: what if he could convince Issa to testify, in exchange for a commitment from the government to give Issa a job and medical treatment?

The ensuing negotiations were complex. Abdoulaye didn't know whether to trust the government representatives and didn't want to be accused of "refusing to cooperate" with them, as he needed their endorsement in order to continue receiving assistance from the agencies. But by confiding Issa's secret, would he be betraying Issa's trust in him? Issa didn't seem too concerned about this. He told Abdoulaye that he would do whatever he could to "help the association" that had helped him; after all, he had nothing to lose since he had been spurned by his own family.

Ultimately Issa did appear on television, but only the back of his head was visible. I watched the newscast with Issa, and he told me this was because he was "shy" at the last minute, and he asked me afterward if it was obvious that it was he who was being interviewed. It is unclear to this day whether Issa ever did get compensated for his appearance—he claims that he did not.

A Second Testimonial Raises Questions

A few months after first meeting Issa, another encounter further troubled Abdoulaye's attempt to forge social solidarities on the basis of a biomedical condition. Matthieu was a Burkinabè who had come from Abidjan and also said he was HIV positive. Matthieu eventually became well known to other Ouagadougou groups that conducted AIDS activities. These groups had always eyed each other warily, perceiving themselves as competitors for the same resources. The case of Matthieu brought them together. From their conversations, they learned that Matthieu was going from group to group, telling a story of illness and rejection and asking for assistance, a prescription in hand. Several groups gave him money to pay for the medicines. Abdoulaye started suspecting that Matthieu was manipulating him, and he inquired with AIDS groups in Abidjan who, it turned out, reported similar experiences with Matthieu. The Abidjan groups had eventually caught on to Matthieu's strategies and refused to give him any more money. It was after this that Matthieu showed up in Ouagadougou, where he was more successful. Abdoulaye explained to me that Matthieu had even managed to get a considerable sum out of government officials when he arrived in Ouagadougou, ostensibly for agreeing to travel to Paris for treatment.

In Ouagadougou at the time, "hustling" was assumed to be the way to survive in the big metropolis of Abidjan, to the south. With over five million inhabitants, the city bred anonymity, and with rank poverty and lurid wealth cheek to jowl, the conditions were ideal for hustlers, get-rich-quick schemes, and improbable spiritualists.[19] Abdoulaye knew this reality only too well, and was therefore more suspicious of Matthieu's claims and more likely to decry them as "tactics" rather than a genuine plea for help. Even though Matthieu came brandishing proof that he was indeed HIV positive—a stamped, laser-printed test result from an Abidjan laboratory—his subsequent behavior bordered too closely on extortion for comfort. Abdoulaye later showed me a letter, written on personalized stationery, that identified Matthieu as a "Licentiate in Occultism and Paranormal Sciences" from the "École Supérieure de Sciences Mystiques (E.S.S.M.) de Lyon" (Lyon Advanced School for Mystical Sciences). He had found it in a pile of papers Matthieu had left at the office. Officially labeled in the African style of administrative French ("Re: greeting. Reference: 006/97/TF/RD/B"), the letter was addressed to his mother. To Abdoulaye the fake letterhead proved that Matthieu was an "imposter" and perhaps fed his suspicions about Issa. Yet Matthieu was not an imposter—his tangible test result and prescriptions would, at first blush, accord him more credibility than Issa, who had only a story. It was perhaps his sheer skill at using the narrative of being HIV positive that first triggered Abdoulaye's doubts about Matthieu.[20]

Meanwhile Issa, after another six months, dropped out of Jeunes sans frontières. In a conversation I had with him in 1997, Issa asked whether I could help him get to Europe. Afterward, Abdoulaye told me that Issa had found work transporting goats on the trains that ran between Ouagadougou and Abidjan. The revelation of Matthieu's strategies and Issa's departure from the group led Abdoulaye to wonder whether Issa may also have been manipulating him and that perhaps he had been "paid off" by government officials to testify. If that had been the case, it would suggest that Issa had not testified solely out of solidarity with those living with the virus but for personal gain and that he betrayed the moral economy that, in Abdoulaye's words and acts, bound together those that lived with the virus.

Concluding Thoughts: On Moral Disruptions

Why, by 1996, were Burkinabè authorities so eager to obtain testimonials of people living with HIV? Testimonials had become, in essence, indicators of success for governments' national AIDS control programs and a key argument in favor of keeping aid money flowing to these programs. Testimonials had become valuable capital for the institutions that could furnish them, and as a result they were prepared to pay. Issa's story—as told by the letter in the paper—was exactly the kind of testimonial the government sought, something that Abdoulaye was not yet quite aware of when he read the letter and invited Issa to join the association in 1995. For Abdoulaye, and Jeunes sans frontières, however testimonials could not be reduced to simple transactions. Indeed, by late 1996, when the search for testimonials was in full swing, Abdoulaye was already caught between two moral economies that were conflated by international agencies' efforts to organize communities with HIV. Disclosure could be valued as speaking the truth of one's self to power and therefore as evidence that "empowerment" programs were successful, or it could be used as a means to foster solidarity. Caught between these two moral economies, it was unclear how to value testimonials. Were they an end to themselves, commodities that could be valued and indeed bought? Or were they merely a means to achieving a broader and more elusive goal, that of organizing communities?

Let us recall how Issa's trust in Abdoulaye was expressed by his "coming out" to him, and therefore reciprocated by his becoming accepted as Abdoulaye's "junior brother." Abdoulaye's flexible use of kinship here reflected how such disclosures were valued as evidence of trust and used to strengthen social ties rather than as items of evidence; paradoxically, it was not the "truth" of the disclosure that was ultimately at stake. Conversely, Matthieu's HIV diagnosis was real and his disclosure therefore "true," but the manipulative aspect of his actions suggested that for him disclosure was not about creating ties. When agencies began to pay for testimonials such as Issa's, they tore them from the fragile social tissue of trust into which Abdoulaye welcomed Issa. They in effect transformed testimonials into a commodity. This disrupted the bonds of trust and disclosure that bound Issa and Abdoulaye. It was therefore possible to interpret Matthieu's actions as motivated purely by financial gain. By negotiating as Issa's advocate, Abdoulaye delicately tried to bridge two conflicting moral economies, attempting to ensure that Issa would get something for his testimonial. Ultimately, Issa left (although it seems that it was not because he felt betrayed). Afterward Abdoulaye told me that he began to doubt that Issa was HIV positive at all. He told me that, after a while, he found Issa "strange" and that the story he told in the letter didn't "make sense" to him anymore: "Africans wouldn't treat one of their own like that," he told me. Abdoulaye wondered whether the story was really true, whether he was used, whether it was _his_ trust that was betrayed.

These stories illustrate the disjuncture between the response of the international agencies and those of local individuals in the early years of the epidemic. In 1994, anxious to "break the silence" and "put a face to the epidemic," international agencies unwittingly created a market where stories about being HIV positive could be bartered for access to resources. This disrupted existing moral economies that had linked disclosure, trust, and social belonging. The narratives that emerged ranged from explicitly sought-after testimonials for formal public events and awareness-raising sessions to stories told to others in search for help with a prescription. Over time, as I will explore in the following chapters, these narratives would take on a life of their own in these matters of life and death, paradoxically pitting people against each other in the name of solidarity and helping to triage those who would gain access to life-saving resources from those who would not. In the next chapter, I continue the story by turning to examine how agencies responded to the paucity of testimonials by using innovative strategies to incite people to disclose. The "confessional technologies" that NGOs and activists brought to Africa generated unexpected effects as they traveled from the cities of America and Europe to villages in Africa.

CONFESSIONAL TECHNOLOGIES

. . . .

Conjuring the Self

[handwritten margin notes: "wld you that? / ever du ds? / w/ other ds? excepti'l / or i's AIDS"]

[handwritten margin notes: "crtnly ther a lot of stories about ppl w/ dis in US ↳ Different culturally? or also incentvzed?"]

[handwritten margin notes: "AIDS = so privte, wrd to in cult / dsclse"]

I want you to close your eyes and to think of someone that you love very much—think of him, think of all the good times you've had together. Think of him, and tell yourself now, "I've got AIDS. I've got AIDS. I've got AIDS!" Think of him, and think of how you've got AIDS. Now, open your eyes. Take a piece of paper and draw a heart. In that heart, write what is in your heart now, when you think of this person you love very much, and then give the paper to your neighbor on the right.

It's early in the morning, 1996, the second day of a meeting of African AIDS NGOs, and Theresa has been asked to do a "warm-up" exercise for the group. Her delivery is dramatic, almost frightening. Theresa is a project officer from the head office of a large funding organization in Washington. She told me later she made up the exercise on the spot "to get people into the feel of things." My neighbor, on my left, gave me a crumpled piece of paper that I never opened. I was so uncomfortable with the exercise that I didn't fill out my heart. Theresa never did tell us what to do with the tiny hearts we all received; after about a year I mailed it back to the shy woman who had given me hers.

I'm going to hand out six of these yellow Post-It notes. Now, think about your work doing community support for people with HIV. Take three of the Post-Its and write a word which expresses what your fears are about this work. And take the other three and write your m̲o̲t̲i̲v̲a̲t̲i̲o̲n̲s̲.̲ Now, one by one, everyone should come up here, share your words with the group and stick them on the appropriate flipchart: this one is for "fears," and this one is for "motivations."

One by one, the workshop attendants place their words on the flipcharts, reading them out as they do so.

Fears
Enough. Tired. Suffering. Suffering. Fragility. Exhaustion. Powerlessness. Suffering. Death. Inability to save from death. Patient confidentiality. Getting overwhelmed. Spiritual and physical suffering. Rejection by society. Lack of psychosocial support. My limitations. Support. Patient resources. Dying. Interruption. Telling the truth. Contaminated. Lack of resources. Suffering. Difficulty to approach. Fear. Economy. Suffering. Pain. Limits. Rejection by others. Fatality. Money. Availability. Disease without a cure. Propagation. Public's ignorance. Pain. Not being up to it. Pain. Discouragement.

Motivations
Compassion. Will to help. Vocation. Personal. Worrisome reality. Support. Pursuing an option. To serve. Helping others. Overcome. Compassion. Useful. Knowledge. Solidarity. Compassion. Fears. Anguish. Help. Love. Help save. Helping others. Overcoming sickness. I could be sick. Comfort. Help. Comfort. Support. Help. Despair. Abandoned. Suffering. Suffering. Love. Be useful. Suffering. Abandon. Spiritual need. Compassion. To serve. Ignorance. Fear. Solidarity. Concerned. Difficult situations. Contribution. Regrets. Love. Hope. Discover myself. Friends who are affected. To l̲e̲a̲r̲n̲.

My neighbor is Aïssatou, a young mother of two. Aïssatou joined a group for women with HIV six months before, after several bouts of illness that led her doctor to test her for HIV. He was the one who recommended that she join the women's group; for him, recommending her to the group was a way to offer her r̲e̲s̲o̲u̲r̲c̲e̲s̲ ̲f̲o̲r̲ s̲u̲p̲p̲o̲r̲t̲ and c̲o̲u̲n̲s̲e̲l̲i̲n̲g̲ he felt he couldn't offer. Aïssatou was selected by the women's group to come to the counselor-training workshop because she was better educated than most of the women in the group.

The funding agencies were taking seriously the lesson learned from the response to the AIDS epidemic in the West: those most affected by the epidemic were best placed to respond to it. What better, they reasoned, than to use HIV-positive people as peer counselors? The workshop's goal was to train lay people to counsel others coming for HIV testing. Its audience was a diverse group of people with HIV who had surreptitiously been referred by physicians or other groups (although their diagnoses are supposed to be confidential) and others who had been drawn to the movement for largely personal reasons.

Aïssatou tells me that she feels that her husband has "withdrawn" from her since she told him the news. He is often away on business. The only person she can talk to, she says, is her doctor. He has been available to her in a way that is unusual for most local physicians. Physicians working in Africa see enormous numbers of patients and tend, perhaps unconsciously, to prioritize those with "treatable" illnesses such as malaria or gastroenteritis. She recalls that he spent fifteen minutes with her when he told her the diagnosis, even hugging her at the end of the appointment, and has twice made an effort to see her ahead of the queue when she has traveled to see him with her concerns. Aïssatou and I met through a mutual friend, Catherine, who had introduced us so I could offer Aïssatou advice on her illness.

Catherine was also at the workshop. I had first met Catherine a few years before, when she was still a social worker at a medical research center in Burkina Faso that was evaluating AZT in the prevention of mother-to-child transmission (often referred to as "PMTCT") of the virus.[1] The center had a long and illustrious history, having been the headquarters for colonial infectious disease eradication programs throughout French West Africa since 1944. As a result, it was the logical place for housing the few AIDS clinical trials being run in the area. Catherine's professional exposure to AIDS was as a counselor to the pregnant women who were enrolled in the trials. After an illness prevented her from continuing her job, she set up the organization as a "gesture of thanks" to the women with HIV, her clients at the center. Their visits and support during her own illness, she told me, had been enormously important to her, and she credited them with helping her to regain her health. The new organization aimed to offer "psychosocial support services" to women with HIV. Catherine told me she had been disappointed that the research institute had been unable to continue looking after the women who had found out they were HIV positive through the clinical trials program but were subsequently determined to be ineligible to take AZT because of anemia.

By the time of the workshop, Aïssatou and I had known each other for long enough to gossip about other workshop participants during breaks. It was initially through our gossiping relationship that Aïssatou came to confide in me. Her worries about her health had led her to borrow money from her family so that she could start a small business on the side: she invested in a small gas stove which she used to fry plantains to sell. "It's not glamorous," she said; after all, she was lucky enough to have had a good education and graduated from high school with the Baccalaureate, "but it's a little something." That little something was almost three dollars a day, which she saved to pay for medicines. Her two girls were five- and seven-years-old at the time, both healthy and precocious.

At the workshop, Aïssatou's yellow post-its ("Lack of psychosocial support," "Spiritual and physical suffering," "I could be sick") appeared to express her experience of her condition in a way that she would never have put into spoken words. She remained silent throughout the workshop, except during the warm-up exercises, which, as one facilitator noted, weren't as "solemn" as the post-it exercise. During these games we threw a ball, played a form of musical chairs called "fruit salad," or sung songs. Nothing personal was involved.

Technologies of the Self

Perhaps the most striking aspect of the response to the AIDS epidemic where I worked in Africa—and it seems throughout the developing world—was that although almost nothing was happening on the ground (clinics were empty, pharmacies bare, and prevention was limited to the broadcasting of public service announcements), workshops, seminars, and training sessions devoted to HIV and AIDS multiplied from the mid-1990s on. I focus here on one workshop, of many I attended, in order to highlight two crucial aspects of efforts to organize communities with HIV. First, the workshops were critical sites of interaction between local volunteers and international consultants who otherwise spent the rest of their time holed up in five-star hotels. In the workshops a hypothetical equality existed between participants. In this liminal zone it was possible to witness processes of conflict and accommodation as people otherwise separated by massive social inequalities—not to mention geography—briefly came together. These were also sites where techniques were deployed to get people talking: what Hunt (1997) first called "confessional technologies." As we shall see, these technologies would have effects far beyond the workshop setting, transforming participants and those around them.

The confessional technologies I analyze in this chapter evoke what the French philosopher Michel Foucault has called "technologies of the self." He points out how, in classical times, philosophy extended beyond a system of thought to comprise a series of practices, including spiritual exercises, dietetics, and forms of self-control. Foucault defines these technologies of the self as practices that "permit individuals to effect by their own means or with the help of others a certain number of operations on their own bodies and souls, thoughts, conduct, and way of being," the purpose being to transform the self in order to attain "happiness, purity, wisdom, perfection, or immortality" (Foucault 1998, 18). According to Foucault, technologies of the self are used to achieve the good life; that is, their goal or telos is an ethical one. These technologies "work" on an "ethical substance," which Foucault defines as "the way in which the individual has to constitute this or that part of himself as the prime material of this moral conduct" (Foucault 1985, 26). As a result, they produce a "mode of subjection," which Foucault describes as "the way in which the individual establishes his relation to the [moral] rule and recognizes himself as obliged to put it into practice" (Foucault 1985, 27; both citations are from Owen 1999, 600). Foucault's definition is useful here because it focuses attention on two important aspects of these confessional technologies. First, they fashion a *substrate*, the raw material of the self: what Foucault called the "ethical substance." Second, they produce a particular relationship of the individual to his or her self—in this case, one that links confession, truth, and the quest to achieve the good life. This is a "mode of subjection" that is directed toward an "ethical telos."

Before his death, Foucault had begun to investigate how Christian confession gradually became a technology of the self. He defined confessions as "a ritual of discourse where the subject who speaks corresponds with the subject of the statement; it is also a ritual which unfolds in a relation of power, since one doesn't confess without the presence, at least the virtual presence, of a partner who is not simply an interlocutor but the agency that requires the confession, imposes it, weighs it, intervenes to judge, punish, pardon, console, reconcile."[2] In this observation, Foucault points out that confessional technologies are also political technologies, reproducing forms of power between individuals and "agencies" that require the confession.

The techniques used in the workshops functioned similarly to what Foucault has described. These confessional technologies instantiated a relationship to an inner self that could be examined, prodded, and told. This is not to say that Aïssatou, Catherine, or I were somehow "selfless" prior to the workshop. Rather, as I will make clear, these technologies made an inner self available in new ways, to me and to my informants, as a *substrate* that must be worked upon: Foucault's "ethical substance." The workshops equipped participants with powerful tools by which they could transform themselves and others. Before describing in further detail how these confessional technologies worked, it is important to understand the context in which they were deployed.[3]

Workshops

The workshops, or "talking shops," reflected the shift away from large, centralized infrastructure development projects—such as building dams—to a more participatory form of development assistance that has championed "appropriate technologies" and small-scale programs that aim to "involve local communities." The explosive growth of workshops indexed the shift from a top-down development model to a more participatory, bottom-up approach.[4] Crucial to this strategy has been the widespread adoption of a partnership model, whereby major aid donors partner with local and international NGOs to implement interventions, in effect outsourcing important pieces of development programs. One widely shared goal was to get locals to "take ownership" of interventions. In the interests of "sustainability," and mindful of the rapid turnover in programs and priorities, donor agencies expected beneficiaries to ultimately assume the costs of programs they were funding. This shift to a more decentralized model echoed global changes in industrial production that resulted in an emphasis on flexible post-Fordist production, outsourcing, and an increased reliance on contractual labor to achieve more "nimble" corporate structures. This implicit emphasis on individual responsibility and suspicion of the state as an actor in development is consonant with neoliberalism.[5]

With this shift to a more collaborative model, workshops became a central component of international agencies' activities in the field. They were a fundamental element of development agencies' programs and a significant component of their budgets, usually under the rubric of "technical assistance" carried out by consultants.[6] Workshops were the key site for interaction with local partners—NGOs and community groups such as Jeunes sans frontières. They aimed to teach the skills necessary to implement the programs and served to monitor their progress once they were underway. For the local partners, workshops were occasions for ensuring renewed funding, as well as for scouting out other opportunities for support. For the local participants, the workshops provided a little extra money, as they were paid to attend. This was a significant bonus in an era of structural adjustment, when many civil servants were paid derisory salaries, if they were paid at all. Per diems (daily expense allowances) for attending workshops could make up the significant part of a civil servant's or an NGO employee's salary, especially when the per diems paid were at UN or international agency rates (enough to cover an international-class hotel). Local participants stayed with friends or relatives and used the difference to supplement their income.

The advent of a flexible model of NGO-driven development meant that most development agencies did not invest in infrastructure or social programs and were often required to rely on paid consultants because precarious funding made it impossible to hire local paid staff. Thus, from a strictly economic point of view, workshops were an ideal vehicle for development interventions, as they were far less expensive than programs that directly addressed the material needs of target populations. Limited to the cost of airfares, consulting fees, per diems, and hotels, workshops generated few unexpected expenses, and once they were finished, they did not generate any ongoing costs. Furthermore, workshops contributed to development agencies' credibility in two ways. First, they were counted as "program outputs." Workshops counted as an indicator of program implementation (for example, "train one hundred village outreach workers"), so that every workshop proved that the program was carried out ("one hundred village outreach workers were trained at a workshop"). Second, workshops helped development agencies collect more qualitative evidence of program success. This could be presented in the glossy reports they produced to justify funding. The photographs, boxed case-studies, and testimonials that figure in development agency reports were usually gathered at workshops for the simple reason that head-office staff and paid consultants did not have the time to travel out to isolated villages to collect this evidence. Let us now return to the workshop to examine in greater detail how these confessional technologies came to be used and the work that they did.

Asking Questions

Most of the workshop was dedicated to training Aïssatou, Catherine, Salifou, and the other participants chosen from other community groups funded by the Washington organization in techniques for looking after the HIV-positive people who come to them for help. This was referred to as "care and support," a term that emerged after several years of linguistic haggling within international NGOs. Theresa's Washington boss, Juan, explained to me that the term "treatment" was "too medical," pointing out that the "medicalization of the epidemic" had been one of the most significant barriers to activism in the early years in the West. With his use of the term "medicalizing" AIDS, Juan meant that doctors, bureaucrats, and other "experts" had been left to manage the epidemic, an approach viewed with suspicion by AIDS activists like Juan. Juan's move to Washington marked a shift from volunteer work in a French AIDS organization to a paid job in an international AIDS organization. But his mistrust of AIDS experts stayed with him.[7] Juan's suspicion of medicalization was shared by activists from other Western countries, such as the United States, where activists blamed government and medical inaction for the deaths of people with HIV.

Being able to communicate with HIV-positive people was a principal goal of the workshop. Participants concentrated on learning "active listening" techniques: how to ask open-ended questions (such as "How does that make you feel?"), reformulating a statement ("When I fall ill, no one will look after me"), or suggesting a response ("You're afraid of being abandoned"), all while mirroring their interlocutor's posture. All this was to build up confidence, in order to "reassure your interlocutor and prove to him that you are really there."

Ask the person you are helping how she is feeling.
Of course, asking just "Are you OK?" is not enough. The person you are asking can answer with just "yes" or "no."
You can ask her, "How are you feeling?" She can then answer that she is feeling well or unwell, and then continue to express herself.
But it is better to ask "What are you feeling?"; "What are your feelings?"; "How are you emotionally?"; etc.
And it's even better if you can link each emotion or feeling she expresses to something precise: "How did that make you feel?"; "What are your feelings about that decision?"; "That's a difficult situation to be in—how do you feel about that?"; etc.
It is preferable that the person you are helping responds by truly describing her emotions—she should be encouraged to speak in her name, in the first

person. For example, if she says "They are telling me that I am depressed," encourage her to say what she really feels.

What counts is not what others say, but what this person truly feels: avoid thoughts which interfere with the expression of feelings, for example:

"I think I am exhausted"

"I feel like I am getting discouraged."

It is preferable that the person be able to say:

"I feel very depressed"

"I feel full of hope today."

The techniques employed in the workshop had themselves traveled from the United States, where they had been developed by social psychologists working for the U.S. military in the wake of the Second World War. Initially designed with the aim of building cohesion within military units, they were subsequently refined in a quest to facilitate racial integration after the Second World War, before being taken up by business schools to train future managers. Ultimately, they would migrate to the counterculture movement before arriving, thirty years later, at the workshop (Lee 2002). In addition to the warm-up exercises, there were "trust-building" exercises, such as having one person stand in the middle of a circle with their eyes closed. She would let herself go limp and allow herself to be tossed around and caught by other members of the group. Pairs or groups of participants practiced their "communication skills" (active listening techniques) using drills: "Ask nothing but open-ended questions for three minutes, then switch. When the time is up, have each member debrief on what the experience felt like."

Participants did role-plays in front of the group in order to practice their interviewing skills. After each role-play, the actors would be debriefed: "How did you feel during the exercise?" Members of the audience were asked to observe the body language and the techniques the actors used. Care was taken to avoid overt criticism of actors' techniques; conveying an attitude of "non-judgmentality" was important.

Ensuring Flow

As a facilitator, Theresa played a key role. The workshop had been designed to fulfill its objectives according to a script not unlike a musical score. Indeed, the script was impressively detailed—each session had thorough notes of what was to happen and was calculated down to the last minute. Post-Its, flipcharts, balls, and the other material supports to the workshop were carefully inventoried and prepared beforehand. Theresa likened her role to that of an orchestra conductor—she only had to follow the score, "reading" the participants the way a conductor would "read" her musicians. In her description of the importance of "distributing speech" evenly among the participants, so that "they should all have a voice," Theresa suggested that the *materiality* of the workshop extended beyond the Post-Its and flipcharts to embrace the *process* itself, which could be sculpted and handled as if it were thing-like.

The facilitators attended a debriefing session every day after the workshop was over. At these meetings, Theresa dealt with the problem of unduly timid or disruptive participants not in terms of personality or personality judgments but as "factors" which needed to be dealt with mechanically. Theresa knew of Aïssatou's seropositivity; she spoke of the difficulty of having to "steer" discussions she thought might be difficult for Aïssatou—notably about death and dying—in such a way as to be sensitive to Aïssatou's perceived fragility, without at the same time making it obvious to the others in the group that this was being done.

Theresa's orchestral metaphor was borne out by the fact that the facilitators did not evaluate the success of the day's sessions in terms of compliance to the elaborate detail of the schedule. Rather, discussion circled around issues of emotional tone and "flow":

> The participants are starting to unwind; I think the warm-up worked very nicely.
> It's a good sign, I hardly had to call on anyone, the discussion circulated nicely among the participants.
> Aïssatou seems less timid today, I think she's starting to process the material better.

A script aided the work of the facilitators. The elaborate pedagogical plan had been worked out on an Excel spreadsheet, with rows allocated to each chunk of the workshop divided according to theme, and columns allocated to objectives, methods, activities, materials, and so on. Facilitators adjusted the spreadsheet every night, based on the conclusions of the meeting; they abridged sessions or modified them according to facilitators' perceptions of what had worked or needed tweaking for the desired effect to be achieved. The debriefing meetings and the spreadsheets showed the workshop's *materiality*. The workshop contained finite quantities of "discussion" to be parceled out as distributed speech; every participant had a voice quotient to be met. Silence was greeted as failure. The participant's psyche contained an emotional content to be "processed" through the workshop, the results of which were legible in terms of how the participant "engaged" with the material: was she still "too involved" or did she achieve some distance? As a result, facilitators could juggle the spreadsheet to achieve the right results. The workshop was inherently *workable*.

The most difficult challenge of the workshop was what Theresa called "maintaining boundaries" and "knowing when to let go." Participants mentioned that they found it odd that they were being trained to encourage their charges to speak of their affliction while simultaneously "not taking it to heart." As this concern became apparent, Theresa introduced a new concept—"setting boundaries"—to aid the participants, and this was written into the script at one of the debriefings. Theresa chewed on a pencil as she presented her idea: she was worried that such talk of "limits" might be "too negative." The title of the exercise was eventually amended to "boundaries and resources." Exercises were developed to get participants to reflect on what their "boundaries" were and how they would know when they had been reached.

Of course, not everything could be scripted. Role-plays could go awry, or an exercise could fail. Participants often brought up difficult interpersonal situations they had faced, such as counseling a bereaved relative or a worried mother. I asked Theresa how it was that she always seemed to know how to advise the participants on what to do in these specific situations. "My experience on the phone line," she answered, "means that I've actually encountered every one of these situations, or something very much like it. All I have to do is recall similar situations and think of what I did that worked best. There's never a right answer—you just learn with experience, what the best things to say are."

Calling, Collecting, Changing

The Brussels AIDS help line where Theresa had volunteered was similar to help lines in other big cities. Callers rang up on a toll-free line and were connected to a volunteer who answered their questions and offered supportive listening. The office was set up like any other call center, with banks of phones and computers where calls were registered and information gathered. A panel display high up on one wall indicated the number of calls waiting, and the number of callers who hung up.

Like the other volunteers who worked at the help line, Theresa had gone through a training workshop similar to the one she was now running in Africa. She had learned the same techniques, using the same vocabulary and the same drills. During the debriefings with the workshop facilitators, Theresa often shared her experiences at the help line. She recalled that most of the calls were fairly repetitive—people would call up anxious because a condom had burst, or requesting apparently straightforward information about HIV and the way it was transmitted. In those cases, skillful use of the listening techniques would quickly reveal the motivation behind the call. Anxious callers worried about the risk of having caught a sexually transmitted disease would admit to an unexpected sexual encounter, or a crescendo of guilt would emerge after a caller divulged the details of a one-night stand. At the time, in Belgium, information about HIV had already been widely disseminated, and so Theresa attributed these urgent dial-up needs for information to "guilt attacks." These calls peaked at regular times—weekend nights or Monday mornings once spouses worried about a fit of infidelity had reached the office and were out of earshot. At those times, the incoming call indicator would glow bright red, indicating a backlog of calls and signaling the volunteers to be as expeditious as possible.

Other calls were "more challenging," Theresa explained to me. A few came from regulars that the volunteers soon enough became familiar with: Theresa characterized them as "lonely hearts," people who had no one to talk to and would call up the AIDS help line "just to talk—you know, Brussels can be a pretty lonely place." At first they made up stories, "perhaps because they felt that if they didn't have an HIV reason to talk to us we would hang up on them." Theresa suspected that they also called up other help lines, such as the suicide line or the psychiatry line, with different stories tailored to fit these lines' particular specialty. These were the most challenging cases because "they couldn't be managed with a simple intervention—you know, counseling, referral, closure." Some of these callers could be "quite manipulative," "laying guilt trips" or even threatening suicide should the volunteer taking the call appear too brisk or dismissive. While the "lonely hearts" represented a challenge because they required quite a bit of skill to handle successfully, others were more emotionally difficult. These were the occasional calls from people with AIDS in moments of personal crisis. Sometimes, people with AIDS would call for medication information; this was easy as it was a simple matter of referral to the doctor on call. But the crisis calls had to be handled by the volunteers, and it was the skills required to deal with these calls that Theresa had come to Africa to impart.

Theresa told me the training was "fundamental" to her ability to deal with the calls; it provided her with a repertoire of techniques to use in dealing with callers. While she too had been trained in a workshop much like the one she was now organizing, her phone-line experience had exposed her to an enormous volume of calls that also contributed to her skill. These calls represented a relatively limited number of situations, much in the way that staff at an airline call center deal with only a small number of situations, despite the large volume of calls: making a reservation, purchasing a ticket, inquiring about the schedule for a particular route, and so on.

Theresa is a sensitive and caring individual, and this clearly played a significant part in her ability to offer support to the phone line's callers. But Theresa claimed her actual effectiveness in achieving "results"—discerning the true motivation of the call, orienting the caller to another resource, delivering the appropriate advice—derived from her repertoire of techniques, or, as she put it, her "skills." The workshop was thus referred to as a "skills-building" workshop. And clearly, her skill derived from her having been able, at the help line, to use different approaches on a trial-and-error basis and from having determined, from that experience, which techniques were effective. If the training provided her with a repertoire of techniques, on-the-job experience allowed her to experiment with a range of approaches so that she eventually became skilled at generating narratives from her callers: narratives of infidelity, of worries, of loneliness.

In this sense, telephone help lines were social laboratories, sites of both control and experimentation that produced experiential knowledge and practical skills. Here, sophisticated telecom systems and techniques of active listening were a confessional technology, collecting and centralizing narratives of distress, and in the process purifying them of any social content. This is analogous to the way hospitals sort patients by diseased organ system, and the way they train health care workers to learn by doing. As a confessional technology, the help line produced capabilities, such as Theresa's ability to know what to say. It also shaped the subjectivity not only of callers, who sought reassurance or advice in moments of vulnerability, but also of operators like Theresa, whose mastery of the skills they acquired there inflected their interactions with others, and even their social relations, in novel ways.[8] Like the workshop, the help line was a material confessional technology that operated symmetrically, transforming the subjectivity of both caller and listener. The central issue for Theresa was how to transmit her skills to her African interlocutors. The ease with which Theresa was able to move and adapt her helpline experience in Europe to the workshop in Africa shows how these confessional technologies were highly portable and therefore could easily be moved across widely different settings.

When Technologies Travel

Despite the materiality of the workshop and its contents—post-its, flipcharts, exercises, techniques, and spreadsheets—it too was an eminently portable affair. Like many other workshops, this one was moved from Brussels to a number of West African capitals in commercial aircraft, with the facilitators sitting in the cabin, and the binders, post-its, and flipchart stand stowed in the cargo hold below. The techniques employed in the workshop had themselves traveled from California, where they were first used in the mid-1980s. In those early years of the epidemic, AIDS organizations trained volunteers to work with people with AIDS: keeping them company, helping them negotiate doctor appointments and hospital tests, even assisting with everyday chores. These volunteers were called "buddies." The volunteer system continued in North America and Europe, even though demand decreased through the 1990s as social services adapted to the problems people with HIV faced, and new effective combination therapies dramatically reduced illness and mortality of people with HIV.

As the effectiveness of antiretrovirals became manifest, the need for HIV companions in San Francisco and Brussels, or New York and Paris, declined. But from 1996 onward, the buddy model swept into Africa on a tide of rhetoric about "sharing experiences." The support of Juan's Washington agency for "sharing experiences" reflected the consensus in the development industry in general, and among organizations attempting to address the AIDS epidemic in particular, that successful interventions needed to be reproduced rapidly to have an effect on the growing epidemic. The term "international best practice" emerged as the key articulation of this consensus by 1997.[9] But to qualify as "international best," practices had to be applicable in different settings; that is, they had to be portable. Certainly, the exercises and drills used in the workshop were portable, as were the techniques used to convey them. Asking questions that cannot be answered by a "yes" or a "no" is a technique that can be used anywhere. However, as became increasingly clear to Theresa during the workshop, getting people to elaborate after being asked open-ended questions was difficult. Laconic answers proliferated. It was difficult to get participants to further develop their answers, even to the open-ended questions. This frustrated Theresa — in this case because it meant there was little "material to work with" in her training sessions. Theresa never asked herself whether, once outside the workshop, the yield of the listening techniques might be just as meager.

The monotony of the answers suggested that there were "technical difficulties." Despite their portability, the techniques, once used outside the workshop, collided with a dense local economy of ideas and practices of the self that in fact interfered with their seamless transfer from North to South. The nature of these technical difficulties was twofold. First, the gaps, evasions, and circumlocutions reflected participants' reluctance to talk about personal difficulties. For them, talking would not solve problems that lay elsewhere, in the difficulties of their material circumstances and the social relations around them. Second, the techniques made certain assumptions about the relationship between questioner and respondent that did not hold up in this local setting. For Theresa, asking questions with "good technique" was a sign of caring, a way of demonstrating "empathy." However, showing "empathy" is a social relationship. As I will discuss below, the notion of empathy attributes a moral value — caring — to a particular social interaction, here, that of asking questions. In the workshop, it was assumed that applying the technique of asking questions would construct a social relationship of caring. This assumed that questions are asked in a social vacuum, which was not the case. The workshop participants were always already embedded in preexisting social relations when they returned to the "field." These social relations, and the material circumstances in which they occurred, meant that applying the imported techniques did not necessarily translate into empathetic local social relations. As a consequence, participants resorted to other techniques to construct a caring relationship.

Lost in Translation

The workshop stressed "attitudes that favor communication in the helping relationship"; one of these was empathy, which the workshop manual defines as follows:

Empathy is neither antipathy nor is it the sympathy we may feel for someone who is dear to us.

It is trying to feel and think what the person we are listening to feels and thinks; it is trying to see the world from his point of view, AS IF we were in his place. But we must never forget this AS IF: because we are never in the other's position.

Empathy is the attempt to totally understand the other, without referring to one's own values.

I had an argument with Theresa about the meaning of the word "empathy." It seemed to me that the definition offered was not correct, that empathy was precisely not about the *AS IF*. Theresa's response was not semantic but practical. She had joined the Brussels AIDS organization after her brother was diagnosed with HIV. She had encountered the term at a workshop in Brussels when she was training to become a counselor on the Brussels AIDS help line. She had learned the term in translation. The term, she told me, came from a humanistic school of psychology founded by the American psychologist Carl Rogers.[10] The organizers of the Brussels workshop had themselves trained in the United States, at one of the original AIDS organizations in San Francisco. The point, she forcefully reminded me, was that something was needed to "maintain boundaries," so that counselors would neither get overwhelmed with the emotional distress they would face, day and night, on the help line nor respond defensively with damagingly judgmental statements like "Why did you do that?" Mobilizing her own experience, Theresa translated empathy into a set of practices for making sure the workshop participants would take home the *AS IF*.

Aïssatou was called upon during the workshop to propose a situation for a role-play to practice empathy skills. It concerned a young HIV-positive woman who was upset by her visiting in-laws' disrespectful treatment of her. In the role-play, another workshop participant, Salifou, counseled the young woman. Salifou had been instructed to practice the new communication techniques. Afterward, the group was asked to "debrief" by commenting on Salifou's use of the techniques and his body language, considered markers of his ability to express empathy. Aïssatou passively observed the role-play she had proposed and didn't offer any observations on how her role-play had been acted out.

At the time, Aïssatou lived in a small one-story concrete house in one of the city's sprawling suburbs. It was when I paid a social call to her there, a few days later, that she introduced me to a gaggle of brothers-in-law who were staying there in her husband's absence—he was away traveling on business. By then her five-year-old daughter, Aïsha, was getting used to me and came to sit beside me as we exchanged greetings. After a while I realized that the scenario she had proposed for the role-play a few days earlier perfectly described the situation she was now quietly complaining about to me. Sisters-in-law had come and criticized the state of the house, and she felt as though her husband had deposited his brothers there to "keep an eye" on her. When I mentioned this to her, she told me that she had offered the scenario as a way of getting advice without implicating herself.

A year after the workshop, Aïssatou had saved enough money from selling fried plantains to open a phone booth. A significant initial investment was required to build the booth and purchase the phone, the small meter for calculating the cost of calls, and the deposit with the phone company. But the phone booth was far more profitable than the fried plantains. "And it's cleaner too!" Aïssatou pointed out to me when she showed me the installations, clearly more cheerful and expressive. The new income enhanced her autonomy but most importantly earned her new respect from her in-laws. And the phone allowed Aïssatou to call a handful of friends abroad whom she had met through the workshops and other meetings she had attended. Aïssatou hoped that her intensified contacts with these Westerners meant that they would be able to find a treatment for her since they presumably would have more access to medications. She confided to me that she was still having problems with her husband. For Aïssatou, then, the kind of talking the workshops emphasized did not provide a solution to her marital and material circumstances, but the workshops did give her access to powerful foreigners and the skills to convince them to help her obtain medicines.

For another participant, the effect of the workshop played out differently. Cicely, a robust church leader and health care activist in a northern town, organized her own workshop after she left Theresa's. She translated the workshop into the national language, Mooré, and used it to train volunteers in her neighborhood association, the Friends of Life Association. The Mooré word they used for empathy, Cicely told me, translates back as "making other's problems your own business." The "friends" also found the techniques useful and had the added advantage that Cicely's unflagging determination had netted them a substantial stock of medications from Europe.

Aïssatou's and Cicely's stories constituted differing strategies for translating "empathy." For Aïssatou, what was at stake was gaining economic independence from her husband and building up a network that could support her should she fall ill. Although she understood and could use the techniques demonstrated in the workshop, she told me she never did make use of them afterward. Nonetheless, the workshop allowed her to develop connections that did eventually translate into access to medicines. Similarly, while Cicely's translation of empathy did not reflect the sense that Theresa had given it, it was nonetheless well adapted to the practical work of her volunteers. They did, in fact, make other peoples' problems their business, by going around and doing home visits. But after all, Cicely pointed out to me, "in Africa, everybody sticks their nose into your business—what's wrong if one takes advantage of it to do good?" The problem Cicely and her volunteers faced was that good deeds were measured in terms of relief from symptoms, not in stories told. She too was able to use contacts that came out of the workshop to obtain medicines. But it was never enough, she told me. Cicely was able to translate the vocabulary of the workshop, but more importantly, and like Abdoulaye had done, she was able to translate the social relations she constructed at the workshop into tangible benefit for her association's clients.

Listeners Transformed

Even if notions of self-help and empathy were sometimes lost in translation, the techniques mastered during the workshop were nonetheless put to use. I learned that this sometimes had a remarkable effect on the trainees, as in the case of two initially shy participants, Jean and Paul. Jean was a catechist from a remote rural area, who had been identified by the funding organization several months earlier. Washington had sent consultants charged with finding community groups that would be able to do "care and support" work. Jean was the leader of a small group of catechists that performed home visits to people who were ill, presumably with AIDS. The "parish companions," like others in their village, assumed that those who were persistently ill or bedridden—most often those who had come back from the city—were suffering from "the evil of the century" (the local euphemism for AIDS).

Jean and his compatriots had been inspired to do this work by the head of their parish, a young Italian priest who had become notorious in the region, and in the Catholic Church as far away as France, as somewhat of an

AIDS crusader. Father Giuseppe, as everyone called him, had developed educational tools—in the form of pamphlets and a game—which stressed that the only way to be safe from AIDS was to be either celibate, faithful, or use condoms. He was later repatriated to Italy. It was said that this was because he had not shied away from promoting condoms, which are forbidden by the Catholic Church. He told me he left Africa because his mother was ill.

Father Giuseppe's departure left the parish companions groups leaderless. When the consultants from Washington came, Jean was eager for an opportunity to "reenergize" his group's efforts. The Diocese seemed uninterested in the parish companions, who nonetheless continued to visit their charges without being completely sure of what they should be doing. The offer from the Washington consultants was quickly taken up, and Paul, a "companion of the ill" from another parish who was also a clerk at the Diocese, traveled with Jean to the workshop.

The presence of doctors, nurses, and other "people of the profession," as they called professional health care workers, intimidated both Jean and Paul at the workshop. Although both were literate, they had never pursued their studies beyond middle school and hence did not consider themselves to be "intellectuals" like the others. On the first day of the workshop, Jean confided to me that he did not know how someone like him, who was not "of the profession" and did not have any scientific knowledge, would be able to understand anything having to do with such a medical topic. In the first few days, Jean and Paul were clearly uncomfortable, and their performance in the various role-plays was wooden. But the workshop's emphasis on drills and practical skills appeared to pay off. By the fifth and last day of the workshop, both Jean and Paul would confidently ask open-ended questions during the drills.

Jean's and Paul's enthusiasm for the workshop actually increased with time. Washington was eager to nurture their investment in the parish companions and provided more consultants to ensure that they maintained their skills and would pass them on to their fellow parish companions. As they attended successive workshops, Jean and Paul changed. They had left the first workshop with a mechanical ability to ask open-ended questions; by the third workshop, they summarized mock interviews with ease and had shed their previously stiff habits to skillfully mirror the postures of their mock interviewees.

The portability of the techniques learned in the workshop allowed them to travel beyond the capital, which served as a stepping-stone in an improbable journey from California to Europe to rural Africa. This happened as those trained in the workshops returned to communities in out-of-the-way places. I kept in touch with Jean and Paul, who lived quite far away from the capital, and when I traveled at their invitation to visit them, I discovered that they continued to use the techniques with surprising effect, even in a place, as we shall see, where life was precarious and famines and epidemics of rapidly fatal diseases were all too common.

The village where Jean lived lay in an arid region in the interior of Burkina Faso; the paved road ended one hundred kilometers before reaching Doumla. On the edge of the road that passed through Doumla was a small wooden stand with a dozen recycled glass bottles of various sizes, which glowed amber from beneath the parasol that shielded them from the bright sun. As a gasoline trader, Jean traveled weekly to the nearest big town, which was also home to the Diocese, to purchase a barrel with which he replenished these bottles. These trips enabled him to maintain a direct line with the Diocese, a link that also enhanced his position as a catechist in the village. Doumla, because of its position on the road, was an important village in the area. It even had a small primary health care center, staffed by a nurse from the Ministry of Public Health. The dispensary was rudimentary, equipped with a few instruments for bandages and a tiny pharmacy that was most often devoid of medicines.

Since Doumla lay in a drought-prone zone, the health of its inhabitants was precarious. The town had never been struck by famine, but many of the village's children were clearly chronically malnourished. As a result, it was not surprising that epidemics of infectious diseases such as measles would regularly sweep the village, killing many of the younger children. The village was also twice devastated by meningitis epidemics, which killed scores of villagers. At the Diocese, I met Catholic nuns who worked in a dispensary linked to the Diocese down the road. They had been in Doumla at the time and told me of bodies having to be "carted away in trucks." They told me that these deaths had never been recorded by the public health authorities. The nuns attributed this to local officials' embarrassment at not having been able to prevent the epidemics. Vaccines and medications to combat the disease had never made it to the village, even though they had been made available for that purpose in the capital; no one was sure why.

Meningitis deaths are quick deaths, unlike those from AIDS. "With AIDS," said Jean, "people lie ill in the family courtyard until the family can no longer afford to care for them." Families would pitch in to buy medicines for ill family members; but when family members continued to be ill despite the use of the medicines, and family resources were exhausted, it was blamed on the "evil of the century." Jean told me that he had seen cases of families who "abandon" their ill—not by casting them out but by leaving them without food or even clothing. He explained this was a case of rationing scarce re-sources, devoting them only to those who are likely to live. As a place where famine and epidemics struck regularly and health care was almost nonexistent, Doumla's inhabitants were thus daily engaged with a struggle for life. The slow unraveling of health that came with AIDS, however, allowed the companions time to step in, to visit and bathe the sufferer and "restore his dignity." Jean was worried about the companions becoming identified as an AIDS group. If that happened, their visits would carry the burden of stigma to their charges.

New Ways of Asking and Telling

In a village where everyone knew everyone, as well as the degree of relatedness between everyone, it might appear odd for the companions, who were not kin, to visit a sick person. This initial hurdle was sometimes a problem, Jean admitted to me, although it was surmountable most of the time because "everyone is used to Church people going around and visiting ill people." The Catholic Church had been active in the region since the 1920s, when the first parish was established. The Diocese still had dusty notebooks that provide a glimpse into life at the mission in its early years: details of visits to neighboring villages, totaling conversions by name and religion of origin, minutes of parish meetings, report cards evaluating native catechists in training, with comments such as "a good boy—hardworking, honest," "serious," "not bright but earnest."

As their home visits continued, Jean's initial worries about stigmatizing those he visited abated somewhat. When I recalled his concerns, he noted that "in a way it doesn't really make a difference," as everyone "knows already." I had asked the question after the companions had already had a year to use the open-ended questions they had learned. The public health nurse in the village, Ishmaël, who had not attended the workshop but had learned of the new techniques from Jean, could barely contain his excitement when we discussed the results of the workshop. "It has transformed the dispensary" he told me. Now that he had begun to ask open-ended questions, "the patients are more at ease." Formerly "laconic," now, "they are talking." I asked what they were talking about, what this meant. "They talk about their problems: money, family problems." What difference has this made? "They have to confide, in a way they never confided to me before . . . it forces them to have confidence." When I asked what this meant for their health, Ishmaël pointed out that health is a "vast thing," that even though there were still no medicines in the dispensary and the patients did not have the money to pay for medicines, they were "relieved" that they had been able to share their problems; and that "counts for something" too. This trust might translate into patients coming for care earlier when they are sick, which meant that their illnesses might be more treatable—assuming they could afford the medicines.[4]

Jean noted that the techniques had given the companions new "access" to the ill. "The families resisted home visits; now they are brought around to gain confidence." He told me of previously distant fathers who have become attached to him and of a woman who confided intimate problems to him, "which in our culture a woman would normally never confide to a man." One hundred kilometers back down the dirt road, at the Diocese, Paul reported the same phenomenon. He even began using the techniques outside of his work with the companions, in his regular job as the parish secretary. "Parishioners come to see me about all sorts of problems, like establishing birth and death certificates, including deaths that have happened in Côte-d'Ivoire." These deaths in Côte-d'Ivoire triggered Paul's suspicions, as "that is where the sickness comes from," and this furnished one of many opportunities to ask more questions. Invited to confide in the parish secretary, the parishioners appeared to do so willingly. "It helps them," he said, and allowed him to feel that he was doing a better job.

Jean and Paul were able to learn and apply the techniques because they were already embedded in social relations where it was expected for them to ask questions. Local people allowed for behavior that could be considered meddlesome from catechists or Diocesan clerks because these were people in positions of authority. When Jean and Paul asked questions, people answered readily because they felt they had to in order to get favorable treatment or gain access to the resources of the institutions Jean and Paul represented. I realized that these techniques for facilitating disclosure between care-seekers and caregivers translated perfectly for Jean and Paul, who worked within an institution where confession was mechanically linked to salvation. Although these techniques could be traced to 1980s California or the consciousness-raising 1960s in America, this was perhaps only a small part of a much longer history that had seen them migrate out of the confessional and into everyday life. Reflecting back on Cicely, Aïssatou, Jean, and Paul, among others, I realized the workshop was a node in a much vaster network which diffused these confessional technologies.

Confessional Technologies

When I followed up with workshop attendants in Ouagadougou over the next year, a somewhat different story emerged. Medicines had become more accessible in the city than in the countryside, and patients more readily assumed that the person who was coming to enquire about their health was a medical professional, rather than, for instance, a missionary. The urban workers were confronted with their inability to supply what patients wanted most: medicines to alleviate suffering. This led some of the workers to hand out symbolic quantities of medicine: three tablets of metronidazole for diarrhea, for instance. (A normal course would require six tablets a day for ten days.). Or they would prescribe tests. Although the results would not lead to any improved chances of treatment, at least it gave the impression that "something was being done." To "stand by" and "just ask questions" would be "just doing theater," the workers said.

They perceived me to be allied with the outsiders who had brought in the workshop. As a result the participants I interviewed and followed were careful to praise the workshop. "It was empowering," they noted, to be able to use and teach the various techniques and to have "shared experiences." But over and over, the problem of material need came up. "These people have treatable illnesses, yet there is no money for medicines," they noted. The donor based in Washington had made it abundantly clear that, while sympathetic to the need for medicines, it would not be possible to pay for them on any systematic basis. "Programs have to be self-sufficient: funding could run out next year, and then what would you do?" Washington intoned, "This is about development, not charity."

A striking feature of confessional technologies was their ability to transform social relations, as those trained to use them observed. These transformed social relations—as when patients began confiding to Jean in the village—in turn changed the listeners. Central to this process was a notion of a "self" that was either revealed through disclosure or transformed through practice. It was a material relationship to the self that became available through these practices—a relationship that had been mute until the deployment of confessional technologies allowed it to be assessed, spoken about, tinkered with, and refined.

Workshops were important sites for translating transnational institutional discourses—like the Greater Involvement of People with AIDS (GIPA) initiative discussed in the previous chapter—into practical, local interventions. The work of translation relied on confessional technologies that could be transported across different cultural environments and were able to produce effects that could be taken up in local networks of practice and signification. Workshops gave me a privileged glimpse into how international consultants and local workers interacted, shedding light onto how differences in opinion, goals, or strategies were reconciled or elided. Theresa's translation of empathy, from its Californian formulation to Ouagadougou via Brussels, suggested why these techniques were so powerful. They worked in both directions to transform the subjects and objects of their implementation, fashioning selves and through them new kinds of social relations. Fine tooled in the laboratory of telephone help lines, they could reliably produce desired effects both in intervener and intervenee.

Furthermore, as we have seen, confessional technologies were strikingly portable. The techniques for "favoring communication in the helping relationship" (the role-plays, the open-ended questions, and so on) were easy to carry from America to Europe and on to Africa, and they worked everywhere. In fact, one European AIDS consultant described to me his fledgling attempts to develop an "international program" in Africa as the "transfer of community technologies." In addition to being portable, these techniques were reproducible. Drills, role-plays, and trust-building exercises played an important role in making the self available as a substance that could be worked on. Workshops and training stabilized the effects these technologies produced across different individuals and different cultural environments. Open-ended questions generated answers and trust, as Jean and Paul discovered. These effects appeared to confirm the reality of the "self" to which confessional technologies claimed privileged access. These artifacts would prove robust as they demonstrated their effectiveness in transforming social relations and indeed the self.

Concluding Remarks: What Did Confessional Technologies Do?

While testimonials were meant to encourage people living with HIV to come out into the open and give a face to the epidemic, they also produced a tissue of disclosure whose fragile bonds could be breached by well-meaning efforts that, by turning testimonials into commodities, disrupted a moral economy. People were trained to testify and encourage disclosure through the use of confessional technologies. As these technologies migrated from the HIV workshops into the everyday lives of those trained, they brought about changes in practices of listening and telling, along with the social relations in which these were embedded. This highlights their potential to introduce new social practices, anchored by a powerful notion of an inner self, beyond those initially intended. Testimonials and confessional technologies, deployed in the context of the fight against the HIV epidemic, encouraged new forms of being and experience whose implications are only now beginning to be explored as they spread more broadly throughout Africa.[11]

Technologies of confession disseminated practices of disclosure, initially in the self-help groups but also, as I learned through discussions with workshop participants, in intimate relations. Several told me that the techniques helped them disclose their HIV status to family and friends. Others confided in me that they in fact used them in everyday relationships with loved ones and that this had in fact made a difference in those relationships. If the training could actually get people living with HIV to disclose their HIV status, perhaps it could also help to make the epidemic "real" and change behavior as a result. However, the migration of confessional technologies out of the workshop could also lead to unintended effects, as we shall see in the following chapters. As disclosure proliferated, it created a social laboratory, where people could experience and learn from the effects of disclosure on those around them.

As I attended discussion groups from 1995 on, I saw previously shy or even taciturn individuals transformed into confident and outspoken people. Thinking about Abdoulaye's confusion as he tried to assess the truth of Issa's and Matthieu's testimonials, I realized that whether the intimate disclosures incited by efforts to combat the epidemic offered a view onto the secrets of the soul, or whether they were a form of "theater" learned through rote and discipline in a workshop, what was ultimately at stake was not the "truth." In the next two chapters, we will see how confessional technologies generated charisma in those who mastered them and how they gave rise to "talking groups" in HIV community organizations. These talking groups then became a passage point in the quest for therapy. As we will see, testimonials could conjure a mysterious substance called "the self" into a powerful life-giving force.

SOLDIERS OF GOD
....

Together and Apart

Many attributed Abdoulaye's success in founding and expanding Jeunes sans frontières to his charisma, and I have found that most of the community groups that emerged in the mid-1990s in West Africa had a charismatic leader at their head. But Abdoulaye never talked publicly about himself, nor was he a particularly gifted speaker. His powers, like those of other activists who emerged at the forefront of African efforts to fight the AIDS epidemic, lay elsewhere, in his ability to broker powerful narratives of conversion, such as Issa's testimonial, into new forms of self-definition and solidarity.

But was this "self" called forth through the use of confessional technologies really new? After all, the religious idiom of conversion in which the testimonials were often couched hearkened back to an earlier history of evangelism and echoed the twelve-step program of Alcoholics Anonymous. Where are we to locate the tentative forms of solidarity and charisma visible in the entangled biographies of Jeunes sans frontières, Abdoulaye, and the organization's members? Do they reflect the historical legacy of colonial and postcolonial encounters between local and global forces, or are they symptomatic of cultural disjunctures? Did forms of personhood and belonging that never existed before come about with AIDS? And if so, how might they play out over time?

The answers to these important questions cannot be found in the story of Abdoulaye and the emergence of HIV groups alone. We must take a few steps back in history and contextualize the involvement of personal testimonials, charismatic leadership, and association in the contemporary response to HIV. Telling this history now will bring into clearer focus continuities and discontinuities in the ways in which personhood, disclosure, and social relations are entangled before and after the emergence of AIDS in this part of the world. The history I tell in this chapter will help construct a genealogy of technologies of the self and the related forms of social organization that emerged around AIDS. It suggests that while practices of self-transformation existed long before the time of AIDS, highly individualized notions of personhood potentiated the technologies of the self introduced to combat the epidemic. This historical flashback begins almost eighty years before we met Abdoulaye, with the story of another young man. His name was William Wade Harris, and he traveled across Côte-d'Ivoire from his place of birth to deliver a powerful message of change. In the wake of his journey, it is now possible to see how his simple testimonial made possible new ways of life.

Harris was born around 1860 in Half-Graway, a small village in what is now Maryland County, Liberia. At the time of Harris's birth, tensions between American settlers, slaves repatriated by the Maryland Colonization Society, and native Glebo peoples ran high. Liberia was still a young country, founded in 1834 by slaves returned from the United States who named their capital Monrovia, after President Monroe. The returnees saw themselves as civilized compared to the "natives" and zealously set about converting the heathens. Harris himself converted to Methodist Episcopalianism in his early twenties, after returning from two years as a *kruboy* on one of the English trading ships that plied the Gulf of Guinea.[1] After his conversion, Harris preached and worked as a schoolteacher.

In 1910, Harris was sentenced to two years in prison by the Liberian authorities for his involvement in an aborted mutiny that is thought to have been backed by the British.[2] The imprisoned Harris became discouraged and briefly returned to the "fetish practice" of his pre-Christian youth. Once in prison he had the following experience:

> Some time before June 1910 he was awakened at night and in bed—during a trance—was called by God (of the Bible) through the visitation of the Archangel Gabriel who appeared to him spiritually as a man in a great wave of light. He was told that he was in heaven, and that God was going

to anoint him prophet, like Daniel, but of a modern time of peace. This God-destined mission was to consist of preaching, fetish-destruction and Christian baptism. (Shank 1994, 115)

Harris did not serve his full term; he was released later that year on recognizance to an Episcopalian minister. He preached in Liberia for another three years before setting off on foot with two companions to spread his message. They traveled east, into Côte-d'Ivoire, on a mission to bring African nations back to God. Exhorting the villagers they met to burn their fetishes and convert to Christ, Harris attracted increasingly large crowds, including a circle of English-speaking interpreters, drawn from the clerks who worked at British trading posts along the way. The arrival of the white man in Africa, Harris preached, heralded the birth of modern times. An era of peace would be preceded by a great world war. The white man owed his superiority and technical advantage to the worship of the true God; the black man could aspire to enter history side by side with the white man only if he abandoned his worship of the false gods of fetishism. Harris's message took hold and transformed the lands he visited: during the seventeen months that his mission lasted in Côte-d'Ivoire, over one hundred thousand people were baptized, and twice that number abandoned the visible signs of traditional religious practices. Harris and his entourage traveled as far as the Gold Coast before turning back to Côte-d'Ivoire. In the end, anxious French authorities, who had come to fear Harris's sway over the "native" population, deported him to Liberia in late 1914.

New Ways of Life

The French authorities were puzzled by Harris. They didn't know what to do about him. Although Harris was briefly arrested twice on nuisance charges, authorities were on the whole rather sympathetic to him, as he encouraged respect and obedience to the colonial government; they were impressed by the fetish burnings and the orderliness he left in his wake. Harris's ability to achieve these results across an ethnically and linguistically heterogeneous territory suggested that he might be useful to French efforts to impose colonial development policies. On the other hand, his ability to mobilize the "natives" was potentially dangerous. Harris denounced colonial authorities for breaking the law of God by making laborers work on Sundays, for example, and colonial authorities were concerned that this might set a precedent for contesting their legitimacy. Harris's journeying had encouraged "natives" to evaluate and debate colonial practices and policies in light of his teachings, in effect setting up a pan-colonial public sphere. Harris's followers were mainly youth and women, undermining the lineage authority of elders. This had the potential to destabilize colonial efforts at indirect rule that relied on the authority of elders. Governor Angoulvant met Harris and was sympathetic to him. However, even the governor's sympathy was not enough, and an increasingly nervous colonial administration finally sent a commandant to arrest Harris in late 1914 in Bassam. Harris warned the commandant he would die if he arrested Harris. The officer paid no heed to the ramblings of the prophet, arrested Harris, and arranged for his deportation back to Liberia. One week later the commandant mysteriously died (Shanks 1994, 3–16).

That Harris's prophecies—the outbreak of the First World War and the death of the commandant, along with a number of other minor ones—came true certainly added to his charisma. His brief arrests and releases led to rumors that he was able to walk through walls and was immune to French authority. But his converts in Côte-d'Ivoire never heard from him again after his return to Liberia. Although Harris continued to preach in Liberia and then Sierra Leone, this never translated into the kind of mass movement witnessed in Côte-d'Ivoire, confirming the common saying that "the prophet is without honor in his own country." In Côte-d'Ivoire, two more Liberian prophets followed in his wake, trailed by a veritable "epidemic" of religious movements that continued to proliferate even after independence.[3] Not all these figures and movements were prophetic. The "black yam movement" of 1918 seems to have been a quasi-religious form of self-destructive resistance to colonial rule, not unlike the Xhosa black cattle massacres of the mid-nineteenth century in South Africa (Zarwan 1976, Peires 1989).[4]

Jean-Pierre Dozon (1995) has argued that Harris's prophesies cleared away an undergrowth of ideas and practices—so-called "fetishism"—that were ill adapted to negotiating the new colonial order. The vacuum that followed was fertile ground for other ideas and movements to take hold. Catholic and Protestant missionaries who had seen Harris outstrip them in his influence over the masses by several orders of magnitude over a short period of time stepped in quickly to fill the gap, at times literally fighting over converts. Harris's charisma was instrumental to forging a path where others could then tread. Harrism was the first social movement to transcend colonial boundaries in Côte-d'Ivoire, a feat that few other prophetic movements were able to accomplish there (Holas 1954). Elsewhere in Africa, similar phenomena occurred under the aegis of other prophets and churches.[5] The effects of Harrism did not recede once the prophetic outbreak was over. The zones of the new colonial territory that fell under Harris's sway in 1913–15 remained receptive not only to new religious ideas but also to new economic practices introduced with colonialism. Specifically, these were the areas that were quickest to adopt cocoa cultivation and the administrative and familial arrangements conducive to a nascent plantation economy (Dozon 1997). Plantations required sophisticated accounting and planning, as well as a system for guaranteeing large quantities of seasonal labor. Therefore, kinship systems had to be loosened to allow cultivators to exercise claims over their sons or their sisters' sons or, alternatively, to allow sons to sell their labor. Harris's testimonials of his visitation, his prophecy of African modernization, the call to burn fetishes and convert to Christianity, all urged that the old ways be abandoned in favor of the new and opened the way to the adoption of these new arrangements.

While Harris criticized some colonial policies, he did not call for revolt against colonial authorities, despite the considerable sway he held over the multitudes to whom he preached. Nonetheless Harris's prophecy set the stage for the emergence of anticolonial politics. By enabling the introduction of new agricultural practices, a new economic class of African planters could emerge and organize planter syndicates. One of these was Félix Houphouët-Boigny, a young planter whose charisma was a driving force in African nationalism. After founding the Syndicat des agriculteurs africains (African Farmers Union) in 1944, two years later he went on to found Côte-d'Ivoire's first political party, the nationalist Parti démocratique de Côte-d'Ivoire (PDCI). The PDCI then helped to establish the pan-Africanist Rassemblement démocratique africain (African Democratic Congress), which gave Houphouët broad recognition across Africa. Houphouët went on to found the Republic of Côte-d'Ivoire and become its president from independence in 1961 until his death in 1993. His aggressive modernization of the country was widely credited for the postindependence economic boom that earned Côte-d'Ivoire the nickname "Switzerland of Africa" in the 1970s; and even when boom went to bust in the 1980s, he was widely revered. Harris's testimonials of conversion and the force of his prophecy were instrumental in dissolving old ways of life, introducing new religious practices, and ushering in questions of how one's moral and material life should be governed, and by whom.

Harris's story, and those of the prophets that followed in his wake, show

how Côte-d'Ivoire's history was already influenced by testimonials that served to bring awareness of gathering individual and social peril, incite hearers to transform themselves, and offer a powerful promise of redemption.[6] The stories of these charismatic leaders also reveal the unexpected historical and political trajectories that are made possible in the wake of such testimonial practices, even when they are not explicitly mobilized as technologies of the self. They are the historical backdrop against which Abdoulaye and others marshaled testimonials—of being HIV positive, of personal transformation, and of the quest for therapy—to forge new social ties, and they may contain clues as to the directions in which this therapeutic quest may take them. This bears keeping in mind as we consider that efforts to organize communities with HIV through testimonials may too, over time, help to dissolve existing ways of life and introduce new practices for the care of body, soul, and community.

Colonial Associations

Practices of association in colonial times extended to "voluntary associations," or social clubs of various sorts, that sprung up in colonial cities and enrolled Africans under the watchful eye of colonial masters. In some respects, this situation foreshadowed contemporary community organizations, including those organized around HIV. Early anthropological studies of voluntary associations suggest that they also played an important role in mediating colonial experience and furnished a space parallel to that of religion where new ways of life could be experimented with. The origins of these associations are unclear. The first such group registered in West Africa was founded in Cape Coast (Ghana) in 1787 "for social purposes and to establish a school for the education of twelve mulatto children" (Wallerstein 1964b, 88). In French Africa, freedom of association, guaranteed by law in the metropolis in 1881, was not granted until 1946. Until then, all groups were obliged to register with the government, which erected a significant barrier to the development of an indigenous civil society. Some anthropologists viewed voluntary associations as vehicles for adaptation to city life by "natives" who were otherwise "detribalized" by the urban environment (Parkin 1966). However, with historical hindsight, a more convincing interpretation is that these groups succeeded in being vehicles for social change by providing forums for the articulation and adoption of new values and norms more adapted to city life (Anderson 1971; Banton 1965).

Many organizations were structured along ethnic lines, focusing on cultural activities such as "tribal dancing," attendance at family members' funerals, and other social events (Mitchell 1956). In addition to specific activities such as dancing or bereavement, they provided a buffer to the economic insecurity of the city (Little 1962). Membership dues were collected and used to offset funeral costs and occasionally to help out members in need. A significant number were rotating credit associations or "thrift clubs": members would pay in a fixed amount every month, with the total sum collected being paid back to a different member every month. They are believed to have originated in the Yoruba institution called *esusu* (Wallerstein 1964b, 95). Rotating credit associations allowed members to create savings in an environment where it was otherwise difficult to save money. With no access to banks, any capital accumulated was liable to be spent recklessly on the temptations of urban life or, worse, be stolen. These associations functioned on trust, a kind of social capital that was afforded by shared ethnicity (Ardener 1964, 216). These thrift clubs outlasted colonial times and continue to exist today.[7] This persistence points to the historical robustness of associations where belonging became translated, to some degree, into increased material security.

In colonial times, voluntary associations were often viewed as a form of adaptation by "traditional" Africans to the "modern" life of the colonial city. Terms such as "detribalization," "adaptation," and "urban kinsmen" were widely used to refer to their presumed "function." However, anthropologists working in Africa disputed this interpretation for over thirty years.[8] They pointed out that alongside tradition, new practices and social relations could clearly be found. In his classic study of tribal dancing in the mining compounds of the Zambian copperbelt, Mitchell comments at length on the various forms of European dress of the dancers that parodied Europeans. This, he argues, was a form of satire that vented otherwise forbidden resentments at colonial authorities and an expression of collective identity unified in opposition to the European colonizer. Mitchell and others have commented on how these associations imitated European forms of social organization, with seemingly undue emphasis on the distribution of administrative titles such as "president," "secretary," and so on. This, along with the penchant for ostentatious dress, led observers to conclude that the accumulation of prestige was very much at stake in these associations. These early ethnographic studies point to the role these associations played in mediating the colonial experience. Rather than seeing this role as one of "adaptation," these ethnographers explored how colonial mimicry produced a space of irony and commentary, where critical awareness of the colonial reality emerged. Voluntary associations were mechanisms for palliating economic insecurity; they were indeed places of laughter, play, and sociality, but ultimately they were spaces where a form of politics could be fashioned.

This historical context raises the question of whether HIV-driven forms of association are also sites from which new political forms may arise. In Harris's time, testimonials were a powerful call to renounce previous ways and begin anew, and they helped usher broader social transformations that found an echo in voluntary associations. Testimonials, however, were not yet explicitly about the "self." They were omens, garnered from visions such as Harris's, which diagnosed the present, forecast the future, and urged change. On the other hand, an examination of socialities in French colonial Africa shows how forms of personhood did manifest within colonial voluntary associations.

Socialities in French Colonial Africa

Ethnographic data on colonial French African cities is difficult to come by.[9] Much of the information that does exist is based on the writings of French colonial administrators. Ethnographies were a hobby (not unlike butterfly collecting), and the bulk of them, primarily focusing on rural life, were produced during the colonial period. Settlers were only interested enough in "natives" to write about their exotic practices. William Cohen's (1971) study of colonial officers shows how students who entered the École coloniale in Paris to prepare for a career in the colonies consistently exhibited a desire to flee the conformity of France, serve the republic, civilize the "natives," and learn about exotic cultures. The Africans most equipped to enter the conversation, those who had been educated to become clerks and schoolteachers, and hence were referred to as évolués, did not really interest the settlers.

However, évolués were the nucleus of a growing African sociality that centered on clubs and cultural activities; historians have since documented these francophone colonial associations (Tirefort 1983). Among the earliest were African schoolteachers' theater clubs, best known for putting on plays. Initially these plays were written by well-meaning settlers who wished to draw on a tradition of African folklore, and they produced pieces such as *A Marriage in Dahomey*, *The Interview of Samory and Captain Péroz*, or *Return to the Abandoned Fetish*, whose titles belie a certain colonial pedagogy. At first, the troupes played to audiences largely composed of Europeans, literate Africans, and even some curious villagers. Over time, however, the plays became popular with urban Africans who, although largely illiterate, were able to understand spoken French. The practice gave rise to a dissident form of theater of which only oral traces remain. Passages in dialect ad-libbed by the actors provided a space for social commentary. African theater paralleled the emergence of an epistolary sociability amongst the évolués. Friendships forged in colonial schools and then maintained through letter writing, despite postings to far-away towns,[10] nurtured a growing political consciousness.

Sporting clubs were another type of colonial association. Colonial authorities actively promoted them from the 1920s. The observation that many Africans had been deemed unfit for military service during conscription for the First World War provided the inspiration for "improving the natives" through sport. Colonial enthusiasm (and the condition that settlers supervise the clubs) was sufficient to win over European fears that sporting clubs might well foment political unrest. Despite investment in playing fields and rudimentary facilities, however, Africans appeared to have initially shied away from the clubs. They preferred the dancing and bereavement societies that were more congruent to their idea of sociability and, besides, could form discreetly without colonial tutelage. Lack of interest on the part of both "natives" and settlers meant that many of the clubs did not survive. The 1936 Berlin Olympics were a turning point. The highly visible victories of black American athletes led to renewed interest on the part of French authorities, who undertook tours of the colonies in search of star athletes (Deville-Danthu 1992). Sporting clubs came to play an important role throughout the colonial period, this time buoyed by generous colonial funding. Elliott Skinner (1974, 266) reports that competition for funding instilled intense pressure among athletes, causing some clubs to break up as athletes jockeyed for colonial funding. As I will explore later in this chapter, this phenomenon was to repeat itself later on, when AIDS groups and individuals went their separate ways and formed their own organizations to compete for resources.

Voluntary associations continued to flourish through decolonization and modernization, even though colonial authorities often thought they would wither away once the "natives" were "detribalized." Jean-Claude Thoret (1974), for instance, found that youth clubs, with chic English names such as the Famous Brothers, the Princes of Liberty, or the Red-Hot Chili Peppers, proliferated in Bouaké (the second-biggest city after Abidjan) and the surrounding smaller towns in the center of the country in the late 1960s and early 1970s. These youth had been to school, and this was reflected in the mission they sought to realize through the clubs. Thoret's informants in the 1970s told him their goal was to "modernize the villages" through "literacy, self-help and educating the peasantry" (Thoret 1974, 8). This mirrors the postcolonial state's mission of evangelical modernization and prefigures ways in which many urban AIDS groups would later carry out AIDS prevention education campaigns in rural areas. Membership in the youth clubs was based on ethnicity and proven through handmade membership cards, complete with photos and stamps. Dances were open to nonmembers and were occasions for youth returning from Abidjan to show off the latest moves. They were also an opportunity for youthful competition, as members from rival clubs would try to disrupt the dances by picking fights. While charismatic individuals may have been a driving force in some voluntary associations, this appears to have been rare, unlike the case of evangelical and other Christian denominations that sprung up in Harris's wake.

This history suggests that like prophetic movements such as Harrism, voluntary associations sought to position their members within the social changes wrought by colonialism and urbanization. They also show how voluntary associations were in some ways social laboratories, allowing new forms of social organization to be experimented with and to spread. Voluntary associations also exhibited a nuanced and complex response to the realities of colonial domination. This response was neither one of outright submission nor open revolt. Bernard Magubane (1971) argues sharply for a political analysis of voluntary associations. He denounces colonial anthropologists' tendency to interpret the mimicry of the state, suggested by the associations' organizational structures, offices, and even regalia, as "play-acting," pointing out that the reality of colonial domination left "natives" little choice but to assimilate.

Forms of association in colonial times generated practices that could take on political significance. They rechanneled social relations and social forms in ways that can not easily be reduced to ethnicity or modernization. Mimicry, letter writing, community credit, and athleticism were first experimented with in voluntary associations. These were highly mobile practices that, once mastered and redeployed in other contexts, could produce new forms of social relations and even political consciousness.[11] Let's recall how technologies for organizing communities in the time of AIDS may also migrate outside the strict grid of NGOs, workshops, hospitals, and community groups mapped by the international AIDS industry. If these technologies and practices do cross those institutional lines, they may produce unexpected effects in the interstitial spaces in which they settle.

Soldiers of God

Let's return now to Abidjan in 1995, mindful of this historical legacy. What links are there between testimonials, healing, and conversion *outside* of efforts to organize communities with HIV? And what might this tell us about what was going on with groups such as Jeunes sans frontières? The pervasive entanglement of religion and healing in Côte-d'Ivoire's time of AIDS emerges throughout the field notes I kept when I worked as an HIV physician in Abidjan.[12] As I watched patients shuttle between churches and clinics, I became convinced that I would have to learn more about the vibrant religious life that surrounded me. I visited many churches and interviewed over a dozen preachers. The Soldiers of God still stand out as a revelatory example of how testimonial and associative practices can produce new and powerful forms of solidarity. The parallels with HIV groups, which sought to achieve the same goals with similar methods, are striking. But, as we shall see, while HIV testimonials and the Soldiers' administration of prophecies both sought to mobilize the self toward greater solidarity, the results differed.

I learned of the Soldiers of God in an eloquent description contained in a thesis on the subject of religion and AIDS in Abidjan (Péducasse 1996). In 1999 the thesis led me to their headquarters at the corner of avenue 18 and rue 23, in Treichville, Abidjan's most densely populated and oldest inner-city township. As Péducasse explains, the Ministère spirituel des Soldats de Dieu pour la Délivrance du Monde et l'Unification des Églises (The Spiritual Mission of the Soldiers of God Engaged in the Deliverance of the World and the Unification of All Churches) was founded in 1983 by Alouhoussène Fadiga, Lord Canon of God, and his two sisters, Fatou Fadiga Lavri and M'Mah Monique Fadiga, Fatou's junior sister. After Alouhoussène Fadiga's death in 1993, the senior sister, known as the Queen of Mothers, took over the reins of the ministry. I often observed her offering spiritual guidance to the Soldiers in Treichville and other townships of the city by cellular phone from her comfortable villa, in the middle-class suburb of Riviera. During my interviews with her there, it was most often the assistant Kouadio Kouassi who was on the other end of the line and who was charged with relaying her instructions to the Soldiers.

I had the pleasure of several wide-ranging and rambling interviews with the matronly Queen of Mothers in her Riviera house, which, she told me, she had designed herself, as she "dabbles in architecture." These meetings were interspersed with phone calls where brisk and quasi-mystical advice was dispatched: "There are negative vibrations happening there—you must be careful!" Or, "This is clearly the work of the Devil! You must be firm." The Queen of Mothers' biography was unremarkable—daughter of a Muslim Guinean father "of the Susu tribe" and a Catholic Ivoirian mother "of the Appolo tribe," she explained that she was raised Catholic and married and divorced twice "because they [her in-laws] wanted to convert me to Islam." She had two boys and seven girls, and worked for many years as an administrative secretary in the Direction Générale des Grand Travaux, the Major Infrastructures Authority, which as its name suggests, was charged with supervising large infrastructure projects. At my first interview, on hearing of my interest in AIDS, she pulled out sheaves of reports of miraculous cures from AIDS. However, over the course of our discussions, it became clear that the Queen of Mothers was more intimately concerned with her charges' everyday afflictions. She attributed these to constipation due to a diet overly rich in palm butter and cassava. We discussed medical-spiritual collaboration for my patients, and in an ongoing correspondence she continued to remind me that I should not be shy about referring difficult cases to her and that in this age of telecommunications one can always do these things easily over the phone. The Queen of Mothers was more grandmotherly than prophetic and had clearly put her administrative skills learned at the Major Infrastructures Authority to good use in running the mission. Prophecy played an important role in the church not by exhorting converts but by providing the substance of administrative practice.

An Administration of Prophecies

One of the Queen of Mothers' important functions was as "chief auditor" of the prophecies that emanated from adepts throughout the city. The prophecies were collected in neighborhood churches, typed, carefully entered into ledger books, and forwarded to the Riviera house for "verification"; it was never clearly explained to me how this was accomplished. Once this was done, they were dated, stamped, and neatly filed in the Treichville headquarters. The ministry was hierarchically structured, using the city's administrative division into townships to attribute continental names to each parish. Yopougon and

Adjamé were "Asia"; Koumassi, Treichville, and Marcory were "Oceania"; Adjouffou and Port-Bouët were "Europe"; Abobo and Cocody were "America"; and the interior of the country was "Africa." Each continent was presided over by a governor and his assistant and a panoply of technical commissions that attended to questions of economics, accounting, literature, sectoral projects, medical and social issues, and information systems. The Treichville center reflected a concern for proper organization. Forms recording services, number of attendees, and prophecies were carefully tabulated and stacked into neat piles. This administrative office was separated from the main entrance, reserved for spiritual consultations. When I first visited the Soldiers of God, I entered through a small hall, where I found young adepts—"Soldiers"—milling about, and then arrived in a courtyard filled with benches. All around, Soldiers prayed loudly, murmuring, chanting, and hissing.

A Gift from God

I was escorted to meet one of the elders in the consultation room, a small dark room off the courtyard, lit only by natural light that fell in through a slatted window. The elder sat in a large padded armchair with her back to the door, her head slightly cocked and coiffed with a knitted wool bonnet. Across from her was a worn couch where consultations took place. Elder Elisabeth introduced herself. She told me that she was a secretary by profession, and came to the ministry in 1986. Her gifts of prophecy and discernment were revealed to her gradually, and she had been an elder since 1993. She told me of the dream where her gift of discernment was revealed: She was in a hospital, in a white gown, and a white woman also in a white gown came to her, took her dossier, and turned around. The Queen of Mothers ("our president") interpreted the dream and said that it was a signal that the Lord had called her to him. Elder Elisabeth had nine children, and her husband had died—was "called back to God"—in 1996. She was "full-time," she explained, while others were "part-time," including the other elder who had the gift of discernment and continued to be employed in the civil service. Elder Elisabeth lived in Port-Bouët, from where she took the bus everyday to the mission. As my interview with her continued, Elisabeth explained that her gift of discernment meant that she was able to listen and offer solace to those who came to see her. It dawned on me that her ability to listen and offer solace was exactly the kind of skill that Theresa's workshop had tried to impart through confessional technologies.

Elder Elisabeth explained to me that she was not trained as a psychotherapist but that her gift had come from God in a revelation that had allowed her to overcome her own suffering, which was rooted in poverty.

Subjects who had undergone "discernment" would proceed to another room for the "exhortation," a séance of Bible reading where the spirits were exhorted to come and heal the sufferer. Péducasse described undergoing a session of "laying on of hands" during which six women prayed over her while massaging her legs, arms, and thighs. Most consultants, Elder Elisabeth told me, came because they were poor and "don't know where to turn." They also knew that the ministry was occasionally able to help out with a bag of rice purchased with donations from churchgoers. The Soldiers that populated the center were fed lunch every day—a certain incentive to stay with the ministry but also an example of how these social ties were strengthened through a form of solidarity not unlike the rotating credit associations we saw in colonial voluntary associations. Unlike these colonial predecessors, and unlike the Harrist Church, the Soldiers of God fashioned solidarity out of a highly individuated form of personhood. Prophecy, "exhortation," and spiritual healing focused on individual bodies rather than more collective ways of living—pointing to how, in the time of AIDS, personhood was already more individuated than in colonial times.[13]

The ministry, like many churches, offered a limited social security net to its adepts. Minimal needs could be met in times of crisis, and those with gifts—of discernment, for instance—could aspire to a more secure position within the ministry. The ministry enacted a classic model of religious solidarity, organizing around worship a community that was able to redistribute resources, offer employment, and provide succor in the face of adversity. The mission's adepts examined consciousness and expressed the results in the thousands of handwritten prophecies they submitted. These testimonials integrated consciousness into the administrative life of the mission and focused adepts' attention inward. Discernment and exhortation were therapeutic actions aimed at self-transformation. They were technologies of the self.

I came to understand that subjecting prophecy to administrative practices such as transcribing, classifying, and filing enabled the proliferation of this technology of the self. Dividing the city and its hinterland into continents, the mission provided spiritual governance to a world proportionate to its geographic reach, echoing the way international agencies and NGOs organize their mission according to a geographic logic. By using the production and management of testimonials, the Soldiers of God waged combat using technologies similar to the ones international agencies and NGOs disseminated in the fight against AIDS. Unlike the latter, however, practical forms of solidarity ensured that Soldiers would not fear hunger or ostracism. These were powerful tools for staving off the threat that competition and schism might undermine association in an uncertain world where poverty was rampant. As we will see, that threat was quick to materialize for community groups in the time of AIDS.

A Proliferation of Testimonials

When international agencies and NGOs signed onto the 1994 Greater Involvement of People with AIDS (GIPA) initiative, first discussed in chapter 1, they endorsed testimonials as the royal road to empowerment and self-help for people living with HIV in Africa. Based on experience in America and Europe, it was held that this practice could encourage solidarity between people living with HIV and allow them to develop a sense of community that could sustain them through the difficulties of their illness. On the other hand, for those who testified, particularly in a context of widespread poverty such as in Africa, the benefit of making public testimonials was not so much the catharsis of airing a painful secret as the possibility of gaining material help from a benefactor, such as a development agency. For some agency workers, this generated concerns that testifiers might be inauthentic and that self-help groups were engaged in mimicry rather than genuine "empowerment"—observations that echoed those heard during colonial times. For the early testifiers like Jeanne, Dominique, Étienne, Issa, and Matthieu, whom we first met in chapter 1, no clear narrative—whether of empowerment or of inauthentic mimicry—emerged. Yet, as we saw in my account of the workshop attendees in chapter 2, testifying did change relationships around those that came forward, as it did for those who employed them. Turning now to explore what happened to those who publicly testified about their HIV status, it is possible to see how confessional technologies of the self led to unexpected effects, much as colonial prophetic testimonials and voluntary associations also led to unforeseen consequences.

In Côte-d'Ivoire, when Dominique, Étienne, and Jeanne first testified at the national AIDS meeting back in late 1994, and then on television, they did so before any obvious opportunity for material gain would have been clear to them. They told me they just had to speak out. Dominique often described a feeling of powerlessness, of having been left "in the dark" after receiving his HIV diagnosis at the country's only testing center in downtown Abidjan. There was no one he felt he could talk to. This feeling was exacerbated at the meeting, where expert after expert rose to speak about the epidemic. All three witnesses thought, "What about us?" None of them was prepared for what would happen after they stepped up to the microphone and said that they were HIV positive. Although they felt something should be done for people like them, they thought they would be ignored. But they weren't.

The health minister immediately promised them support, in the form of a place to meet at the headquarters of the national AIDS program. Not long after, the invitations to speak came, along with offers of financial help and "technical assistance" to help set up and structure the group as an official AIDS organization. The largest French AIDS organization faxed their constitution from Paris, which was used as a template for a new organization called Light for AIDS, after Dominique's experience of "coming out of the dark." The organization's flowchart, with Dominique at its head, traced an impressive structure: a president, flanked by assistants who in turn presided over a number of *commissions* (committees): *prise-en-charge* (care), *testing et conseil* (testing and counseling), éducation, and so on.

Although HIV testing was not widely available in the early 1990s in Africa, in Abidjan a free and anonymous testing center had been operating since 1994. Together with recruitment efforts by researchers for clinical trials of HIV drugs, this meant that significant numbers of people had been diagnosed with HIV. A number of those people joined the new organization. With the ready availability of Western sponsors in Abidjan, Light for AIDS was able to offer incentives for membership: subsidies for transportation costs to attend meetings and, some hoped, the possibility of a trip abroad to attend a conference. Perhaps because organizational charts tend to be long on structure and short on purpose, what exactly Light for AIDS was supposed to do did not seem clear to many of its members. Discussions with its Western sponsors, who had in mind such model groups as Uganda's highly publicized TASO (The Aids Support Organization), encouraged Light for AIDS to develop outreach activities for the ill and supportive counseling to others who had been diagnosed HIV positive. International donor agencies started subsidizing these types of activities for members of groups such as Light for AIDS in 1995.

More lucratively, group members received stipends to testify about their HIV seropositivity in meetings organized by the agencies to promote AIDS prevention. Typically, a Light for AIDS member would stand up in front of a group of schoolchildren or factory workers or villagers and talk about being HIV positive. The testimonials were most often preceded by an information session where figures on the epidemic, modes of transmission, and the nature of the virus were presented, followed by demonstrations of condom use and question-and-answer sessions. These testimonials themselves often seemed stereotyped. For instance a male testifier would talk about how he too never took AIDS seriously, until—for one reason or another—he took the test and found out that he had HIV. Now, he is wiser, takes care of himself, and always uses condoms. In more intimate settings, some of the testifiers would refer to their condition of knowing their HIV diagnosis as a form of enlightenment. Étienne once told me, "The guys in the neighborhood, they used to laugh at me; they probably thought they would be laughing over my dead body. But now I have traveled—I have seen Europe, South Africa. I have seen something, and they still know nothing." These testimonials' emphasis on the discovery of a "truth" that forever changes the discoverer and his behavior, reminded me of stories about being converted or born-again.[14]

Ventilating

In the eyes of agency workers who shepherded its development at every step, the core business of Light for AIDS was "self-help." For them, Light for AIDS would provide a forum—through the weekly meetings whose attendance they subsidized—where people with HIV could get together, share their problems, and be mutually supportive of each other. Most of these agency workers had met people with HIV in the course of their jobs and had been privy to the difficulties they faced. It was not an easy litany to hear. In Côte-d'Ivoire, as in most developing countries, regular health care is unaffordable, except for a minority with health insurance or the very wealthy. Most of those who joined Light for AIDS had been ill, as this was how they found out they had HIV in the first place. They had had to scrounge money from relatives to pay for an expensive prescription or an even more expensive stay in the hospital. They expected that this scenario would be repeated and knew that the resources would not hold out indefinitely. At the time, the only HIV testing available was in hospitals, although clinical trials for testing drugs to prevent transmission from mothers to children during labor also tested large numbers of healthy women in Abidjan.[15] Some people with HIV had lost their jobs, their spouses, or their children to the disease. Knowing that one had HIV, as one informant told me, was "knowing you are condemned to a slow death and most probably to being abandoned by your family and friends—not because they don't love you anymore, but because they can't afford to look after you and won't be able to bear looking you in the eye because of that."

Faced with the near impossibility for individual staff to resolve these social and medical problems, having a group like Light for AIDS to refer people to came as a relief to the development agencies. "At the very least," said a colleague of Madame Janvier's to me, "they'll be able to ventilate." Dr. Konaté, a French public health physician who trained at the University of California, Berkeley, in the late 1980s and took a particularly active interest in the group, was less sanguine. While in California, she had been impressed by patient activism and AIDS activism in particular, which at the time was just beginning in France. Clearly, Light for AIDS was not quite the same kind of organization. Through frequent and involved conversations with the women in the group, Dr. Konaté had realized that the women "didn't have a voice" in the organization and that they did not feel that the organization was supportive of their concerns. She was struck by how Light for AIDS, and other organizations she worked with in Africa, "mimicked the state" with their "obsession" with vice presidents, task forces, and commissions where nothing ever really happens. "I realized that in many respects it was just an empty shell," she told me, unwittingly echoing earlier colonial dismissals of voluntary associations as only mimicry.

At first glance, the meetings gave credence to Dr. Konaté's impression of postcolonial mimicry and nonaction. They always began formally, opened by the president, or, in his absence, the vice president, followed by reports from members who had attended prevention workshops to give testimonials or had gone to other meetings. Reports were often lengthy and gave the impression of being used to justify the reporter's having done whatever he or she was reporting on. They were most often long descriptions of what had happened, or who had said what at such and such a meeting. Members would begin to talk only at the end of the meetings and then complain about the difficulties of carrying out an activity that they had been commissioned to do. Often, these discussions would become acrimonious, with members accusing other groups, or even one another, of concealing valuable resources. After all, it was no secret that wealthy Western agencies were giving money to the organization, and that the group's president and vice president often had the opportunity to travel to Europe, South Africa, or even the United States. So why, members asked themselves, was the group barely able to afford bus fare to do home visits? And who was going to pay for their prescriptions when they got ill, as was sure to happen through visiting patients in the TB ward or in the filth of the city's shantytowns?

A Minor Incident

The group, along with others, convinced the World Bank to fund a March for World AIDS Day in 1995. The march was from Adzopé, fifty kilometers north, to the center of Abidjan. The bank paid participants to walk and offer testimonials at HIV prevention events along the way.[16] The price of their participation had been energetically negotiated with the World Bank, and the fee of one hundred dollars was settled upon for a fixed number of marchers from each AIDS group. Rumors that circulated about a French magazine's having paid five hundred dollars for interviews with Africans with AIDS certainly served to increase the price. But the first day of the march, more participants showed up than the organizers had expected. A small fistfight broke out between a number of participants over who would march and receive the stipend offered by the World Bank. The march finally went on as planned.

Although news of the fight at the Adzopé-to-Abidjan AIDS March never officially got back to Madame Janvier, funding for a repeat event the next year never materialized. Light for AIDS continued to struggle throughout the next year. Funding was episodic, and matters were not helped by Dominique's illness. Despite this, Dominique went to the International AIDS Conference in Vancouver the next summer, in July 1996. At the last minute an embassy gave him a free plane ticket, so he went on the long trip. But when Dominique got to Vancouver, he did not have money for the conference registration, accommodations, or food. Luckily, he had made enough contacts at previous conferences so that he was looked after. But Dominique was quite ill, and later that year, shortly before World AIDS Day 1996, he died. In death, old rivalries were forgotten. It was a typical funeral: several wakes in the city, followed by a "traditional" burial in his village. What was not so typical was the interest the event generated. Dominique's death was covered in a few local papers, and a large following of activists in different local AIDS organizations attended the wakes and traveled to the village for the burial. At the World AIDS Day parade, marchers could be seen sporting buttons that read, "Dominique we miss you." Jeanne took over the presidency of the organization.

In many ways the organization never recovered. Jeanne never seemed to achieve the legitimacy Dominique had. She traveled often—too often some thought—and a European AIDS organization gave her a cell phone so that they could "get through to her at any moment." Rumors swirled around her: that she wasn't really ill; that she was ill and that witchcraft was keeping her healthy; that she was a witch; that she was a lesbian and a wealthy Belgian lover was keeping her; that her family had rejected her; that she had rejected her family. As these rumors proliferated through 1998, donors made clear their desire to shift their interest to "empowering women with AIDS." One official with a donor agency explained to me that "women with AIDS are the new priority." Many of the women who had originally been in Light for AIDS left to form Abidjan Women against AIDS (AWA).

Thus, between 1996 and 1999, Light for AIDS splintered off into at least five groups, one of which retained the name and some of the original members. Some of these splinter groups were referred to as "one-man associations," ostensibly because they were formed by individuals seeking to access funding from development agencies. By 1999, the mantle of heated "donor interest" had passed from Light for AIDS to AWA. Another group, which was originally set up by missionaries at an evangelical AIDS care center in a poor quarter of the city, had since acquired a reputation for being outspoken. Renamed ACT-UP Abidjan, it drew its name from its Parisian homonym (which is incidentally its main French sponsoring organization), itself inspired by the radical New York group of the early 1980s that pioneered Western-style AIDS activism.

Fission

If Dominique's testimonial was a watershed in Francophone West Africa, the subsequent evolution of Light for AIDS resulted in its consignment to relative obscurity. The story of the group's multiple schisms was unfortunately the norm. Throughout Africa and elsewhere other workers in agencies and NGOs I met reported the same. Even though individuals may have been willing to talk about their experience of illness in public, growing funding from donor agencies raised the financial stakes enough to warrant fierce competition between members for real and imagined access to material resources. A common result was the formation of splinter groups—at times "one-man" or, more rarely, "one-woman" associations—to more effectively compete for these resources.[17] This pattern of schism repeated what occurred fifty years earlier when French colonial authorities began funding voluntary associations; schism generated more conflict.

Abidjan Women against AIDS (AWA) was "adopted" by another, more established organization, Positive Nation. As their name suggests, Positive Nation was one of the more outspoken groups, and it had a platform—in the form of regular radio and newspaper columns—from which to air their views, which were often highly critical of the government. They also had good connections to Abidjan's upper class, as well as a number of local benefactors who had supplied them with a house in the Abobo quarter of Abidjan and an office in a building in the central district of the Plateau. Like Jeunes sans frontières' office in Ouagadougou, the Positive Nation office doubled as both a reference library—cluttered with glossy brochures and lavishly illustrated pamphlets from Northern NGOs and thick reports from WHO and the World Bank—and a prevention and counseling center where the groups' members would relay messages about safe sex, condoms, and loving people with HIV.

The house in Abobo was donated at the same time as some medical equipment and drugs, and Positive Nation decided to make it into a drop-in center for people with HIV. This was not unlike Jeunes sans frontières, which independently opened a "Café solidarité" at roughly the same time. But the medical equipment went unused for two years, as the group proved unable to apply for and obtain funding to actually run a program at the drop-in center. Gradually, as the center accumulated other equipment—a computer, a photocopier, a television with a VCR—from other programs, Positive Nation members from the neighborhood would gather to hang out, learn how to use Windows, or watch African music videos on channel 2. Because the space was largely unused, it seemed logical for the group to offer AWA a space for meetings.

Eventually, one of the group's more entrepreneurial members, Yao, decided that it would make more sense for Positive Nation to go into business rather than waiting for hand-outs from bureaucratic aid agencies. The +Shop opened in late 1998, selling staple items: candies and gum for schoolchildren, biscuits, tinned coffee, milk, tomato paste, soap, sugar, rice. In its selection of goods, the +Shop differed little from other corner stores in Abidjan, except for one important detail: its start-up capital came from donors rather than banks or private investors. Positive Nation's institutional credibility allowed it to raise funds from agencies, and this furnished capital for investing in the new business. The photocopier donated by the UN was intended for reproducing documents for other NGOs, but it was mainly used to sell photocopies to the public.

The +Shop was a huge success, generating enough revenues to employ four people, one of whom was HIV positive and earned a double salary to cover her medication expenses. Yao, always looking for a new project, convinced the group to reinvest the proceeds from the +Shop to set up the +Café: a snack bar that could employ women from AWA. The project was agreed to, and by mid-1999 two thatched gazebos had gone up in front of the house; one had a half-dozen small tables, and the other housed a small kitchen. Yao had succeeded in persuading Positive Nation to invest its capital in two Chinese portable gas burners to heat the large woklike pans (made from recycled palm oil barrels) used to deep-fry plantains, yams, and fish.

AWA's involvement did not turn out to be a success. Initially, none of the women wanted to work in the +Café kitchen. Some said it was because they feel like they "only belong in offices," and they didn't want to "get their hands dirty" frying fish. Others said it was because they felt they were not going to be paid enough. Yet when one of the women brought a cousin from the village to take on the job, the other women accused her of favoritism and hijacking the group's resources. After a few months and only one major glitch—one employee disappeared with the proceeds of the till—the Café had become popular with neighborhood locals and was turning a healthy profit. But the women resented that the Café's profits were being used to pay back Positive Nation's investments—building the gazebos, buying the gas burners, plates, and cutlery. "Why should we work for them?" they asked at increasingly recriminatory meetings. It was during this period that donor interest in AWA heated up. A large Berkeley nonprofit organization, "dedicated to empowering women with HIV," identified AWA as a local partner. It funded AWA to organize home visits where AWA members would "peer counsel" other women with HIV. As is common in these programs, AWA had to account for the grant money it received from the Berkeley organization by submitting reports about the home visits by the "peer-educators" (the HIV-positive women of the group). Few visits were carried out, but deciding who would fill out the reports became the focus of acrimonious debates at the group's meetings.

The dissensions that consumed AWA in 1999 stemmed from an argument over how resources were to be allocated within the group. AWA had come into existence in response to development agencies' desire to fund self-help groups of HIV-positive women. In the context of the desperate poverty in which AWA's women lived, the dynamic within AWA was not one of self-help and solidarity but of competition over resources. It was a question of "what's in it for me," as the Ivoirian representative of their Berkeley funder put it. This attitude was reinforced by the implicit message of the agencies: "because you are HIV positive, you deserve our help." Positive Nation took this message to heart in its sincere offer to help the fledgling group. Many of the women were deeply hurt by the acrimony and bitter exchanges and by what they felt was the injustice of the situation. All the women in the group struggled to get by in everyday life, but stark evidence of injustice stared them in the face every time they met. Some of the women had qualified for a program that allowed them to receive subsidized treatment with antiretroviral drugs, but the program did not have enough space for all the women. Over that year, the women on the medicines gained weight, while those who didn't receive any got thinner and fell ill. Two of them died that year. By then, it had become clear to me that within the groups, members were competing over life-saving medications.

Two Solidarities

Jeunes sans frontières and Light for AIDS, despite their different histories, illustrate a shifting and indirect confrontation between two models of social ties. The international development agencies' promotion of testimonials as a path to empowerment and self-help was rooted in the assumption that solidarity stemmed from disclosure and sharing secrets, not material resources. Discourses such as that of Greater Involvement of People with AIDS (GIPA) as well as the way development officials attempted to foster solidarity among their African charges promoted a specific understanding of "self-help." For officials like Madame Janvier, mutual support is a result of talking, sharing, and discussing one's problems in a nonthreatening environment. In this view, self-help happens as people fluently articulate issues that affect them as individuals, constituting an imagined community where individuals are brought together by their affliction. The testimonial, or public disclosure of one's HIV positivity, is crucial: being able to "come out" in a small group is a small step toward the larger act of "coming out" publicly. Underlying this model was the notion that there is a hidden truth to the self and that when this secret is shared, personal catharsis results and social bonds are formed.

This model of self-help ignored existing networks of obligation, responsibility, and exchange that both constituted persons and bound them together in a different moral economy. This moral economy did not require self-disclosure as a social glue; indeed, such an act was often viewed with suspicion and as a sign of selfishness and lack of consideration. My informants repeatedly expressed to me their fear of being ostracized by their families and their neighbors for talking in public about being HIV positive, and often drew on idioms of kinship to underline these powerful forms of belonging and reciprocity structured around family and community. As a result, Abdoulaye, Issa, and the women of AWA were in a kind of "no man's land" that lay between two moral economies. On one hand, organizing communities of people living with HIV was about solidarity and self-help; on the other, well-meaning efforts to support "empowerment" with much needed material support and confessional technologies of the self fostered competition and undermined trust.

Moreover, at times they found themselves in conflicting and even untenable positions, as the act of disclosure risked alienating them from all-important kinship ties. For them, dissolving these social relations was not an option—for who would look after them after the development agencies left or moved on to new issues? Who would look after their children? Nonetheless, many embraced the possibility that "coming out" might offer much-needed resources. Confronted with the threat of illness, these individuals were open to exploring these new social relations and grasped eagerly at Western models of solidarity even as they were only too aware of how little power they had over their material or social circumstances.

Abdoulaye tried for many years to organize, as he called it, a "groupe de parole" (discussion group) of people with HIV who could come together and talk about their situation. Jeunes sans frontières always expressed its mission in terms of "African solidarity" for people with HIV, and at first glance, it always seemed a logical next step for Abdoulaye to be concerned with setting up a "talking group." But the group didn't get off the ground for the first few years because no one wanted to meet, much less talk—even though they knew that other members were in the same situation. "What are we going to talk about?" or "People will find out" were the most common reasons for not speaking out. The dilemma of Issa's testimonial was only the first incident where Abdoulaye was confronted with the difficulties of translating between these two forms of solidarity. Talking was a social adhesive that did not, at first, stick in a setting where kinship framed the terms of solidarity. With the growing availability of HIV treatments in Africa five years later, as I will explore in the next chapter, coming out about being HIV positive would lay the basis for a novel, biomedical kinship based on a shared condition and the potential for therapy. ← *Hope*

A Matter of Life and Death

Since colonial times, voluntary associations have offered a bulwark of community in growing cities and a chance to participate in the social transformations that concentrate there. They have been places where economic and social technologies are used and mastered, as the examples of rotating credit associations, bereavement societies, or theater clubs show, and they translate into concrete forms of solidarity. Despite similarities in forms of association and in reliance on social technologies, community groups of people with HIV differ in one striking aspect. In a setting of pervasive poverty, where biomedical care for illness is largely unaffordable, being diagnosed with HIV dissolved any stable sense of the future. When people with HIV came to community groups, their concerns were a matter of life and death.

The perceived dangers of disclosure made resorting to kinship networks dangerous; whether family would support the patient or turn away was not always clear. Disclosure is perilous, as Issa reported in chapter 1 when he sought support from his family in 1993. On a daily basis, families confronted illness and had to ration scarce resources for care. The American medical anthropologist Nancy Scheper Hughes (2003, 206) has called this "lifeboat ethics," the equivalent of deciding who must be sacrificed so the others may live. Hein Marais, who has written extensively on South Africa's AIDS epidemic, points out that we are not all bobbing around in the same boat (Marais 2005). Community groups were boats adrift amid the wreckage of a burned-out state, survivor communities wed by the ambivalent potential of a strange biomedical kinship.

I began this chapter by drawing a historical parallel between Abdoulaye and the prophet Harris. Abdoulaye never claimed to be a prophet, and indeed would scoff at such a comparison. However, in his ability to marshal testimonials of conversion such as Issa's or Étienne's to leverage new social relations based on a shared biomedical fate, I suggest that Abdoulaye and other activists share a common genealogy with prophets such as Harris. When Harris swept across Côte-d'Ivoire prior to the First World War, the territory had just been conquered by a hostile and foreign power, and those that survived huddled in villages and towns facing an increasingly uncertain future. His testimonial of conversion and the prophecy that resulted offered a narrative of salvation. As Dozon (1995) explains, it was also a powerful technology that helped introduce new ways of life that laid the groundwork for an independent republic to emerge less than fifty years later.

In West Africa's time of AIDS, the Soldiers of God, as well as other churches and faith-based organizations, are able to foster a pragmatic solidarity through scripture and worship. Meanwhile, Abdoulaye translated Western idioms of self-help based on shared affliction and evolving notions of interactive kinship into a pragmatic solidarity. This was not an easy task. As Issa's and Matthieu's stories illustrate, the "self" of self-help (and the notions of authenticity and truth telling it implied) got lost, or at least resisted translation, at times tripping up community leaders like Abdoulaye who found themselves worrying whether telling the truth was an indicator of trustworthiness. Nonetheless, a "working misunderstanding"[18] allowed some measure of resources to flow from international agencies to community-based organizations, and the agencies could claim they were doing something about the epidemic. The effect over time was the emergence of social relations hesitantly organized around the idea that people living with HIV were bound together by a shared fate.

While Abdoulaye was able to translate this into pragmatic form, such that solidarity became a measure of material security, this was a challenge for other groups where solidarities were too fragile to withstand the dynamic of competition fostered by the international agencies. The Soldiers of God, in contrast, were able to use testimonials—prophecies—as a social glue to bind adepts together within a hierarchical mission. Administrative technologies and charismatic religious practices of healing may have focused attention on individual selves, but they were yoked to a practical form of redistribution that bound together adepts, whatever their financial circumstances, and ensured that none would go wanting.

Testimonials were powerful incitements, and their call to renounce previous ways and begin anew recalls evangelical idioms of conversion. In the present case, it is too early to assess whether this potential will indeed result in historically robust transformations. In Côte-d'Ivoire, practices involving conversions, testimonials, and forming associations predated the AIDS epidemic, particularly in times when fate was uncertain. They are precursors to how community came to be organized in the time of AIDS, driven by powerful confessional technologies that addressed the self. Examining these customs sheds light on how linking practices of forming associations and providing testimonials may generate powerful forms of experience. This historical exploration identifies the paths by which these practices have in the past set the stage for the emergence of previously unimagined developments, and it prepares us for the consideration in the following chapter of how a powerful notion of the self would come to be charged with life-giving powers.

Within these early HIV community groups, competition over the resources that began to flow in those years from international funders trumped the fragile sense of solidarity that was supposed to flow from sharing a diagnosis. For some, being able to talk about HIV meant access to life-saving medications or even, in the cases of Abdoulaye, Étienne, Jeanne, and a few others, the chance to start life anew in Europe. Most, however, remained poor, and many died; they were the ones whose narratives did not gain traction and did not translate into valuable social connections. As I will explore further in the following chapter, being able to talk about oneself became a matter of life and death. Under the rubric of self-help and empowerment, a working misunderstanding solidified, such that florid demonstrations of international solidarity were put forth at the same time as discrete mechanisms that determined who lived and who died worked their way into the very fabric of communities living with HIV. It was possible to be both together and apart.

LIFE ITSELF

....

Triage and Therapeutic Citizenship

On Monday, 10 July 2000, South African Supreme Court Justice Edwin Cameron, speaking at a plenary session of the International AIDS Conference in Durban, declared "I am here because I can pay for life itself." This chapter explores how with the discovery of effective treatment for HIV in 1995 and in the continuing efforts to organize communities with HIV, practices of forming associations and providing testimonials reformed around a sharply focused goal: life itself. The material I present here draws extensively on my own experiences as an HIV physician in Montréal and Abidjan, where I was involved in the introduction of the new treatments that revolutionized HIV care. I saw firsthand how practices that had tried to foster and nourish solidarity among people with HIV now helped to separate those who would receive treatment and live from those who would not. This was triage, and this chapter chronicles its emergence. In its wake, a therapeutic citizenship has emerged as the hallmark of a "politics of life itself" that defines the struggle to survive in biomedical terms: a politics of life and death.[1]

A Therapeutic Revolution

In 1995, clinicians in North America and Europe began to see the benefits of what was then an experimental treatment paradigm that relied on combining multiple antiretrovirals (ARVs) in the treatment of HIV infection. The paradigm emerged with the development of a a new class of drugs, protease inhibitors (PIS), which target a crucial enzyme that the virus requires to reproduce itself. Previous drugs had targeted reverse transcriptase, the virus's "signature" enzyme that allows it to transcribe its RNA back into DNA. These drugs are accordingly referred to as reverse-transcriptase inhibitors (RTIS), which are divided into nucleoside and non-nucleoside type (NRTIS and NNRTIS respectively). Protease inhibitors are remarkably powerful antiretrovirals; however, biological resistance to the drugs was found to emerge very quickly, attenuating their effectiveness. As a result, drawing on the success of combination therapy for the treatment of tuberculosis, the idea of combining RTI-type drugs with the PIS was advanced as a strategy for delaying the emergence of drug resistance and permanently suppressing the virus. The strategy and the new treatment paradigm it defined—combating resistance through strategic drug combinations—revolutionized HIV treatment.

By late 1995, HIV clinicians across the industrialized world had all seen dying patients return to health with the new drug combinations. At the Montreal General Hospital, where I attended as an HIV physician, our patients had been dying at a rate of two a week. Within a few years of the new treatments' introduction, only a handful of patients died each year. New viral load tests showed that the drug cocktails suppressed viral replication to the point that HIV was no longer detectable in the blood, and biological tests showed that with treatment patients' immune systems were being restored. The adoption of what came to be called highly active antiretroviral therapy—HAART, for short—had an enormous impact, reducing deaths from AIDS by over half in industrialized countries during the first few years of their use. After fourteen years of bad news, it was almost too good to be true. At the 1996 World AIDS Conference in Vancouver, optimistic researchers debated the possibility of curing patients with the drug cocktails.

Although eradicating HIV from patient's bodies is no longer considered likely, HAART marked the advent of a therapeutic revolution akin to the discovery of insulin for the treatment of diabetes. An illness that was previously fatal, in most cases, within a few years of diagnosis, is now treatable and has been transformed as a result into a chronic condition. It is not unreasonable, given the current state of knowledge, to expect that those people newly diagnosed with HIV will live lengthy and productive lives: a recent Danish study estimated that with access to treatment, HIV shortens lifespan by about twenty years. A thirty-year-old woman with HIV, for instance, can expect to live to be sixty-five rather than eighty-five (the life expectancy of a woman without HIV) (Lohse, Hansen, Pederson, Kronborg, Gerstoft, Sørensen, Væth, and Obel 2007); by early 2010 data had begun to emerge that in the North people with HIV could expect to have a normal life expectancy.

How Activism Produced Treatment:
Clinical Trials and Therapeutic Citizenship

The discovery of the efficacy of these drugs—their ability to suspend the ticking time-bomb of viral replication, restore health, and almost indefinitely postpone illness and death—was itself linked to an earlier therapeutic activism that did much more than exercise direct political pressure on the biomedical establishment to find a cure for the disease. Most accounts of drug discovery focus on the process of laboratory research; however, only a fraction of drugs found to be biologically effective in laboratories make it into clinical practice. In the "real world" of patients' bodies, drugs may prove to be ineffective for a range of reasons: they are too poorly absorbed, cause too many side effects, are too toxic, or are metabolized too quickly. Clinical trials, where drugs are tested in real patients, are necessary to weed out the truly effective drugs from those whose promising results in the test tube won't translate into clinical results.

Recruitment into clinical trials for HIV in the early years of the epidemic in North America, Europe, and Australia was facilitated by a strong therapeutic militancy that was rooted in a decade of gay activism, which generated significant expertise about drugs and biomedical research among AIDS activists and people living with HIV. This was accompanied by a strong willingness to participate as research subjects. This readiness drew on a sense of political engagement in the struggle to find a cure for the disease. Participation in clinical trials demonstrated what can be termed a kind of *therapeutic citizenship.* This politicization of research participation has since spread to other diseases, as has been documented by medical anthropologists who have studied the proliferation of patient self-help groups around specific illnesses.[2]

Today, recruitment is the biggest challenge faced by clinical trials and the pharmaceuticals industry that most often sponsors them. Enormous sums of money have to be invested in recruiting and then retaining patients. Because it takes so many patients to statistically tease out a treatment effect from chance, trials have to be run in multiple sites, most often in different countries and can cost hundreds of millions of dollars. As shown by a number of high-profile failures of "blockbuster" drugs that did not succeed once they were tested in clinical trials, the stakes are enormous not only in terms of the potential health of thousands or even millions of patients but also financially. The cost of failure also raises the financial stakes in recruitment efforts. Ironically, such clinical trials benefit from a kind of therapeutic citizenship born of the activism of the grim, early AIDS years. Volunteering to participate in clinical trials grew out of a sense of duty so that others may benefit from treatments eventually found to be effective. This situation is what bioethicists would call altruism; however, I prefer to examine it through the lens of citizenship because of the activist and political dimensions to clinical trials.

The development of a politicized consciousness, and indeed of a form of citizenship, around HIV was a two-edged sword for pharmaceuticals firms. Most visibly, therapeutic activists were quick to accuse the firms of refusing to make drugs accessible, sparking at times highly visible and embarrassing protests. However, therapeutic activism and its corollary of citizenship also made recruitment and retention in trials easier, potentially diminishing drug development costs. Both continue to inform an ambivalent relationship between the industry and the activists. Quietly aware of the benefit of therapeutic citizenship to recruitment in drug trials as well as public relations and tax benefits, the pharmaceuticals industry funds community groups through "community programs," even as they worry about the potential for activists to influence shareholders and cut into profits. In parallel, activists are deeply suspicious of industry's motives even as they are kept alive by the drugs. Until the mid-1990s, therapeutic citizenship remained confined to the North, as there was no significant research on HIV treatment being carried out in the developing world.

The first major trial that took place outside Europe, North America, or Australia was Merck's 1997 "028" study, conducted in Brazil, comparing triple therapy (using two standard HIV drugs alongside the drug indinavir) against monotherapy (indinavir alone). The study generated controversy (though surprisingly little) because some patients were kept on the single therapy arm of the study long after other trials proved that triple therapy was better and was therefore the standard of treatment. In effect, those in the indinavir-only arm likely developed resistance rapidly to the drug, compromising their future options for effective treatment. Normally, when it is determined that patients in a trial are actually receiving inferior treatment, the trial is terminated immediately; however, this was not done in the Brazilian case for rea-sons that remain unclear (Oliveira, Santos, and Mello 2001).

Another trial, this time conducted in Africa, generated even greater con-troversy. In Africa, while no trials using ARVs to treat patients were conducted at the time, a number of clinical trials were carried out to test various ARV drugs' efficacy in preventing HIV transmission from mother to child (this is abbreviated as PMTCT, for "Prevention of Mother To Child Transmission"). These trials became the subject of fierce debate in scientific circles in 1997. Although AZT had already been shown to decrease PMTCT by two-thirds in previous experiments, these trials tested a simplified AZT regimen against a placebo. Proponents of the trial argued that the placebo-controlled arm was necessary to quickly prove the effectiveness of AZT in developing coun-try settings. Opponents denounced the placebo as racist and drew ominous comparisons with the Tuskegee experiments of the 1930s–1970s. In this in-famous study, African American men with syphilis were never offered peni-cillin, even after it had been shown to be effective in treating the disease, in order to not interfere with the study's goal of describing the "natural" (that is, without treatment) progression of syphilis.[3] A short time later, a PMTCT trial comparing the new drug nevirapine to AZT was conducted in Uganda, which while showing the effectiveness of the drug, became the focus of a controversy relating to the initial use of, once again, a placebo (which was subsequently dropped), as well as its study design, data management practices, and statis-tical analyses.[4] These controversies, however, failed to ignite AIDS activists in the West, for whom, by and large, the issue of access to treatment in the South did not gain any traction until 2000. That was to change with the emergence of an indigenous African activism that, in Francophone West Africa, was in-advertently unleashed by two clinical trials.

How West African Clinical Trials Produced Activists

In the mid-1990s, two large clinical trials of AZT for the prevention of mother-to-child transmission of HIV were conducted in West Africa, one sponsored by the French National AIDS Research Agency (ANRS) and the other by the rival American Centers for Disease Control (CDC). The French study tested 14,385 women in Bobo-Dioulasso (Burkina Faso) and Abidjan, while the American study tested 12,668 women in Abidjan. All the women received state-of-the-art pretest counseling for HIV. Of the more than 27,000 women tested, 3,424

(13 percent) were found to be HIV positive. However, in the American study, 618 HIV-positive women never returned for their results and the post-test counseling, while in the French study the figure was 648: that is, 37 percent of HIV-positive women didn't find out their diagnosis. Researchers told me that the rate of nonreturn for results was lower in HIV-negative women, suggesting that women with HIV suspected their diagnosis and decided not to return for results. Of the HIV-positive women who returned for their results, only 711 (32 percent) were included in the actual trials, the remaining 2,182 (68 percent) women having either been excluded for medical reasons (discussed below), or because they did not consent to be in the trial (Dabis, Msellati, Meda, Wiffens-Ekra, You, Manigart, Leroy et al. 1999; Wiktor, Ikpini, Karon, Nkengasong, Maurice, Severin, Roels et al. 1999).

The trials had an enormous impact in shaping the early response to the epidemic in both Burkina Faso and Côte-d'Ivoire—simply because of the sheer number tested. In those early years, HIV testing programs were relatively few and far between—in the Ivoirian metropolis of Abidjan, for example, there was only one site that provided free and anonymous testing in 1995. In Burkina Faso, there was little or no access to HIV screening, including screening blood transfusions. As a result, only a handful of people knew their HIV status. The few who were tested were often not told of their diagnosis; as we saw in chapter 1, health care workers feared the demoralizing effect that doing so might entail.

The relative lack of HIV testing elsewhere, as well as my own medical experience in Abidjan, led me to believe that the majority of those who knew their HIV status had found out because they were initially recruited to participate in the trials. Of course, only a small minority were actually enrolled in the trials, which needed to screen a very large number to have a significant pool from which to enroll a necessarily smaller number of selected, eligible study-subjects. Women were disqualified from participating in the trials for numerous reasons; not arriving early enough in pregnancy to receive the AZT, and suffering from anemia (which could be dangerously worsened with AZT), were among the most common. Women who had tested positive but who had not been eligible to enroll in the trials complained bitterly to me that they had been "discarded." They resented that they did not have access to the panoply of services offered to the women who had been included in the trials. Indeed, women who were included in the trials did receive medical care and social services that were not available to others.

After having been tested, many women found their way into community groups in search of material and social support. Some even set up organizations for their fellow would-be trial subjects. These women made up the bulk of the membership of early groups of people living with HIV in both countries. Yet, as this account makes clear, the reasons that led them to participate in this clinical trial did not amount to the kind of therapeutic citizenship that drove people with HIV in North America, Europe, or Australia to enlist in clinical trials. It was poverty and fear of the consequences of being HIV positive that made them enlist in the trials in the hope of gaining access to medical care, rather than an abstract notion of solidarity with others suffering from HIV.[5] Nonetheless, within a few years, a more radical kind of therapeutic citizenship emerged from the lack of access to drugs and the work of a few therapeutic pioneers.

Conversion

In late 1997, Abdoulaye traveled to Europe for the first time. He had been invited by a French NGO to attend a workshop there. Traveling to France was enormously exciting—an opportunity that few Burkinabè would ever have. By then Abdoulaye was spending most of his time putting together HIV projects for Jeunes sans frontières. Once in Paris, trips to the Eiffel Tower, the Louvre, and the Champs-Élysées were complemented by visits to the French AIDS organizations whose material Abdoulaye had been reading and whose names were by now important references for him. Abdoulaye took the "exchange and sharing of experiences" purpose of the trip seriously. He visited HIV testing centers and counseling groups that he had read about. He also had an HIV test, which turned out to be positive. Even worse, he had almost no more T4 cells and was classified as having AIDS as a result.[6] Parisian friends found a doctor who was able to supply him with HAART for himself.

After he returned from Europe, inspired by the self-help groups he had seen there, Abdoulaye convened—but did not participate in—a discussion group of people who had come to him because they were HIV positive and had heard that Jeunes sans frontières was involved in the "fight against AIDS." However, at these meetings, no one spoke about being HIV positive. Discussion centered on the details of everyday life and the difficulties of getting by. By 1999, Abdoulaye was faced with a new problem. He realized that some of the people he had invited to the group were better off than others—some of them were even able to pay for some form of medical treatment. This would surely "inhibit" any of the kind of spontaneous discussion that was important to mutual support; he worried at the time that it would "only create jealousies and frustrations."

During the time he was trying to set up the "talking group," one of Abdoulaye's aunts in the family compound fell ill. She had been sick for some time, and unbeknownst to her, she had tested positive for HIV at the local hospital. As was customary at the time, the diagnosis was confided to her father, the head of her household, and he had summoned his knowledgeable Abidjan-educated nephew to discuss the matter. Abdoulaye arranged for medical care and made sure that she was properly looked after and that her medications were paid for. Her diagnosis was never discussed. She died six months later, not having been told she had AIDS. Although I helped care for her, Abdoulaye never spoke to me about the effect her illness and death had on him.

The challenges Abdoulaye faced in starting a self-help group indicate that the process of "telling" and "sharing" was indeed difficult in settings such as these, where sheer poverty could magnify even minor inequalities, lead to jealousy, and undermine solidarity. As we saw with Light for AIDS, Positive Nation, and Abidjan Women against AIDS in the previous chapter, the resulting rivalries and competition tore groups apart, leading to schisms in many community groups of people living with HIV. In settings of numbing poverty, the Western dream of self-help, characterized by perfect sharing and caring, was more illusion than practical strategy. Uncontained disclosure had the potential to upset social hierarchies, such as those in Abdoulaye's family, that had been negotiated over long periods of time.

For Madame Janvier of the World Bank and other Westerners I interviewed who worked to support community organizations responding to AIDS in Africa, it seemed obvious that self-disclosure was cathartic and a first step to the organization of therapeutic social relations. Although Abdoulaye told me he believed this too, this was belied by the different manner in which disclosure occurred around him. While he was encouraging others to talk about being HIV positive, until 1999 he himself never spoke about his HIV positivity or of his worries about those who were close to him whom he knew to be ill.

Therapeutic Solidarity

Early in 1999, Jeunes sans frontières embarked on a new project called the "Friendship Center." As the organization developed a higher profile, local physicians and even the National AIDS Control Program began referring people with HIV. Abdoulaye, inspired by what he had seen on his trip to France, conceived of the Friendship Center as a combination drop-in center and dispensary. The Friendship Center was located in a small house with a courtyard in an outlying neighborhood of Ouagadougou. An erratic flow of medicines from concerned friends in Paris made for a small stock for the dispensary—"nothing much," Abdoulaye told me, but certainly better than what was available at the nearby state-run dispensary, where years of World Bank mandated cost-recovery had long ago emptied the pharmacy.

As the volume of patients grew, an informal camaraderie was struck up in the house's living room, which doubled as a waiting room. It was airier than the organization's headquarters and had two wooden benches, a small table, a shelf full of AIDS literature, a large color television, and a VCR. The TV and VCR had been obtained through a World Bank program. The patients often sat watching the television, exchanging long formulaic greetings as others arrived or left. All of them had at some point learned they were HIV positive, and some were visibly ill. They all knew that the others sitting around them were HIV positive. Yet never, in those first months of operation, did they discuss this situation among themselves.

Things began to change, however, in early 2000. By then, Abdoulaye had been on his antiretroviral treatment for almost three years, managing to get by with donations from his Parisian doctor. Together with this doctor, Abdoulaye had devised a treatment plan to deal with erratic supplies; he would just switch medicines according to what he had on hand, making sure that he was taking at least three different and complementary drugs. He had bought a small fridge to store those medicines that had to be kept cold. As a result, by late 1999 his T4 cells had shot up, from fourteen to over four hundred, and his viral load had been undetectable for almost three years.

He put on weight, regaining the stocky build of his early twenties. His girlfriend Fatou also thrived with a supply of medicines from Montréal, but their daughter Salimata was often ill with fevers. While this is not unusual for a child in West Africa, Abdoulaye was distraught every time she took ill. For the first year of life, HIV tests are unreliable, as infants still have their mother's antibodies at that point. Because Fatou was HIV positive, her daughter Sali would have tested positive too. By the time she was two, Sali still had not had a test, even though at that point it could have been reliably ascertained whether or not she had contracted HIV. By that time, Abdoulaye had resigned himself to preferring uncertainty—punctuated by attacks of anxiety every time Sali had a fever—to the possibility of definitely finding out his daughter had HIV.

Meanwhile, Abdoulaye's visible recovery had an effect on his surroundings. Rumors circulated that he had supernatural healing powers, and this brought a new influx of the ill to the Friendship Center. Those who knew about his consumption of medicines did not suspect HIV, he told me, because he had always been "easy to take medicines," a quirk that his Ouagadougou friends assumed had been acquired in Abidjan. His stock of antiretrovirals did seem ostentatiously modern, laid out in their brightly colored boxes by the foam mattress he slept on in the adobe room in the family courtyard where he lived.

The doctor in Paris was also impressed, telling me that he had "never imagined" that such a striking clinical response could have been obtained with rotating medicines and a long-distance therapeutic relationship. As a result, in early 1999 he began sending Abdoulaye away with armfuls of medicines for other patients in Ouagadougou. By 2000, Abdoulaye was telling some people he was HIV positive but "only my friends who are taking the test or have taken it," he told me, "because only they can understand." That year, he moved out of the family compound. His daughter's frequent illnesses had led the other women in the family compound to accuse his aunt's mother of witchcraft. As I helped him pack up his antiretrovirals in their pristine packages, Abdoulaye told me he was "tired" of these "African stories" and wanted a holiday.

Storytelling and Triage

Faced with the influx of newcomers at the Friendship Center, Abdoulaye tried again to start a "talking group." However, the patients maintained an awkward silence. Discussion invariably turned to the problems of material subsistence. A European psychologist who tried to work with the group told me that these people are "completely overwhelmed by their material needs and difficulties—how can you expect to do any psychological work until these more basic issues get resolved?" But with the arrival of medicines, things began to change. With circumspection, Abdoulaye and an inner circle of Friendship Center staff began carefully—"little by little"—to distribute the medicines.

He explained to me that they used the talking group to identify candidates for the medicines—those who came regularly were more likely to observe the rigorous treatment schedules and those who "contributed" most to the group were favored.[7] These "dynamic" members should have access to treatment, they reasoned, because they would be able to help others more than those who remained passive. The "talking group" began to fulfill a function unintended by those who championed it as a model of self-help: it served as a kind of laboratory for identifying those who should have access to treatment. Thus the self-help group functioned as a triage system, a method for determining who would benefit most from medicines—just as in wartime, when military physicians must decide who among the wounded can be saved and who cannot.

Interviews I conducted with other activists during that period confirmed that the story of Abdoulaye and Jeunes sans frontières was not unique. Many members of community groups involved with AIDS prevention in the mid-1990s were HIV positive. Some learned of their diagnosis before joining, while others did afterward, taking the test (as Abdoulaye did) in order to "practice what they preach." As a result, these organizations, like Jeunes sans frontières, inevitably found themselves drawn into the issue of treatment for their own members as well as for those who came to them for help. Ultimately, access to treatment was contingent on social relations and the ability to capitalize on social networks. Jeunes sans frontières made treatment decisions based on a social calculation: who would translate improved health into the greatest good for others? The few who did get the drugs through this improvised form of triage were initially a minority. Many obtained antiretrovirals through contacts with Westerners. For these individuals, the key to survival was to be able to "tell a good story." Some activists made it to France, where AIDS activists took them in and helped them obtain residency permits. The French authorities, like other European countries, quietly renewed HIV-positive foreigners' residency permits, subsequent to domestic political pressure denouncing early deportations of HIV-positive Africans.[8] Those who stayed behind in Africa viewed those who left as the truly lucky ones—those whose stories had got them to Europe.

Friends who told me they were HIV positive had differing experiences with the drugs. Ange-Daniel never wanted to go on the drugs. He just didn't think he needed them, and he was right for another ten years. He only started on the drug cocktails in 2008. Kouamé became active in a local HIV group, becoming somewhat of a cause célèbre because of his charismatic testimonials of being

HIV positive. His oratorical skills eventually helped him to secure a supply of HIV medicines from a European contact he made through the association. As he became more involved in the group, he confided feeling guilty that he was on medication while others were not. He rationalized to himself that, at least, his being healthy meant he could contribute to getting more drugs for others, which he continued to do for several years. As the supply of donated drugs increased from 1998, however, Kouamé and his colleagues in the group were increasingly faced with the gut-wrenching prospect of deciding who should get the drugs. No matter how many donations they received, demand always outstripped supply.

As already mentioned, the concept of triage was developed on the battle-field, as a way to use scarce treatment resources in the most rational way: those most likely to live are prioritized to receive care, while those whose prognosis is poor are left to die. Kouamé and his group, like most other groups faced with the same situation, made the difficult decision of who should bene-fit from the limited source of drugs by adopting a form of triage. But how did the groups chose? Kouamé, like Abdoulaye, reasoned that those who were most charismatic, most able to deliver effective testimonials would be the best advocates for getting more drug donations. Gradually, over time, this reason-ing subtly introduced another outcome to the discussion groups: what was at stake was no longer "talking and sharing" but the identification of those whose continued health was most likely to translate into increased resources for the group. Sometimes the decision as to who should get the drugs was more directly pragmatic. Prioritizing access to drugs for beneficiaries who would facilitate the group's work in virtue of their professional position, for instance, as a customs officer, was an example of how groups reserved drugs for members they considered valuable.

Over time, those who were gifted communicators also became those with the most direct experience with the drugs. Echoing the experience of AIDS activism in the North, these patients were often the most knowledgeable people around when it came to their treatments. When treatment programs expanded after 2002 in the wake of scaled-up funding for HIV treatment in Africa, they were ideal candidates for assuming leadership roles in the new programs. Others exploited their connections differently. Kouamé managed to get a visa through his HIV contacts to go to France in 2002. Once there, he obtained a permit that allowed him to stay in France "on humanitarian grounds" because he had AIDS. But the permit did not allow him to work legally. When I last spoke to him in 2004, he lived in what was called a "therapeutic apartment" in Marseille that was provided by the French government for those who could not work because of a medical condition. But he was lonely there and talked of starting a new AIDS group for other Africans who were in the same situation as he was.

The Institutionalization of Triage

For Abdoulaye and those that followed the same therapeutic journey, the improved health that came with antiretrovirals embodied the discourses of empowerment that had up to then been limited to a rhetoric of self-help. Affecting groups of people living with HIV, where many sickened and died, the advent of antiretrovirals meant that it was life itself that was now at stake—for them, and for those around them. Their ability to harness social resources to leverage access to the drugs translated into healthier bodies, a biological transcription of the discourse of empowerment. That skill, produced and tested in the disclosure laboratory of the discussion groups, triaged who would have access. For others, however, personal activism was less of a factor, particularly when they were able to obtain treatments through the handful of African pilot programs that began, somewhat piecemeal, in the late 1990s. These programs institutionalized triage under the cover of administrative procedures, medical criteria, and the need to ration scarce resources.

Launched in 1998, the first program in Africa that sought to provide the general population with access to ARVs was a joint initiative between the Ivoirian Ministry of Public Health and UNAIDS. The UNAIDS initiative was a pilot program coordinated by the agency to improve access to antiretrovirals (similar programs were launched in Uganda, Vietnam, and Chile). Its inception reflected the political pressures that HIV-positive Africans and their allies were putting on the agency. True to the rhetoric of empowerment, UNAIDS had cultivated a constituency of HIV-positive African "stakeholders." Simultaneously, people living with HIV across the continent were being trained using the self-disclosure technologies in the kind of workshops I described in chapter 2. This subsequently turned these individuals into effective advocates for an emerging public of HIV-infected and HIV-affected Africans. UNAIDS hired an Irish consulting firm with close ties to the pharmaceuticals industry to negotiate reduced prices for antiretrovirals with pharmaceuticals firms and implement a distribution system in the country. The Ivoirian government pledged one million dollars to a drug-purchasing fund that would be used to subsidize the medicines. Interestingly, UNAIDS did not itself make any financial contribution to drug purchases. According to the officials I interviewed in 1999, this was "beyond their mandate" as a "coordinating and technical support agency."

The program got underway in late 1998, recruiting patients at the Infectious Diseases Service of the Treichville University Hospital, one of the city's TB control clinics, and at a handful of NGO outreach sites. The program quickly became embroiled in controversy. Several hundred people were treated through the initiative; however, the subsidies were insufficient to allow them to afford the recommended three-drug cocktail for more than a few months. Almost all of those who continued could afford only two-drug cocktails. As a result, the majority became resistant to these drugs.

Informants at the American Centers for Disease Control laboratory in Abidjan told me about the irregularity of follow-up, which meant that blood specimens were collected at more or less random intervals, rendering any kind of meaningful epidemiological analysis difficult. It was nonetheless evident in the clinical data I reviewed at the time when I worked in Abidjan that many patients were becoming resistant to the drugs. Prescribing physicians, selected from a variety of public health institutions across the city, had minimal training in using the drugs, limited to a three-day seminar conducted by a French AIDS NGO. I learned this through a workshop on ARV prescription I organized with colleagues in Abidjan in 1999.

The selection criteria for subsidies were never made clear. One group of activists, the splinter group ACT-UP Abidjan, had been quite vocal at the Geneva AIDS Conference in 1998 and was granted an unprecedented 95 percent discount. Its members were therefore able to afford the triple-therapy cocktail with this subsidy. The group ceased to be active on the local AIDS scene from then on, fueling rumors that they had been "bought" with the drug subsidy. The coordinator of the program explained to me that the generous subsidy had been an administrative error. It was never clear what role the drug distribution system set up by UNAIDS with the Irish consulting firm was to play. The prices that had been negotiated by the consulting firm were in fact going market rates, and as prices for antiretrovirals dropped through 2000 and 2001, the program was briefly locked into a higher price.

By 1999 the program quickly became mired in an ongoing corruption scandal that erupted when several billion francs earmarked for health aid from the European Union went missing—a situation that resulted in the suspension of EU assistance to the country. As political and economic problems mounted, the national Public Health Pharmacy stopped getting reimbursed for its ARV purchases. As unpaid debt mounted, its ability to purchase other essential generic medicines was compromised, and discontinuation of ARV purchases ensued. This, combined with poor inventory management, led to repeated stock-outs of antiretroviral drugs. Thus, throughout 2001, the supply was patchy at best, meaning that almost all of those on the UNAIDS program had intermittent, partial therapy—a situation certain to generate drug resistance in the patients concerned. Although patients complained bitterly about the situation, little could be done.

In retrospect, it seems unreasonable to have expected Abidjan's crumbling public health facilities to shoulder the burden of such an ambitious program. Staff in hospitals and clinics complained that they were not compensated for the extra work that the program entailed. Furthermore, after launching the process, UNAIDS did not follow through as enthusiastically as it might have done with technical support to monitor drug procurement and distribution, as well as the training of physicians. However, it is still debated whether the program can be termed a failure—after all, many patients did obtain the antiretroviral drugs.

The fact that tens of millions suffer from AIDS means that hundreds of thousands die every year. This supports the claim that AIDS is a public health emergency, as the UNAIDS Initiative maintained, and emphasizes the need to develop rapid and at times improvised measures to get drugs to people. Yet, HIV is a slow and chronic condition, which means that the benefits of antiretroviral therapy do not occur until after at least several months of treatment. Thus, while the epidemic may be a political emergency, it is rarely an emergency in clinical terms. That is, unlike a heart attack (which requires treatment in a matter of minutes to save a life), HIV infection does not cause immediate death, and treatment does not immediately save a life; rather, it prolongs survival, as long as treatment continues. Paradoxically, it is HIV's relatively indolent but inevitably fatal course that enabled therapeutic citizenship to arise. This happened as people diagnosed with HIV transformed into activists who demanded access to treatment, articulating their claims based on the official declaration of a state of emergency.

The Biology of Triage

For treatment activists, therapeutic citizenship was *embodied* as the drugs restored health—stark evidence that it was life itself that was at stake. The social factors I have described here as triage, which resulted in inequalities of access to the drugs, were transcribed into a biological difference between those that got treatment and those that did not. Triage can also lead to more subtle forms of biological differentiation, as drug use changes the virus itself. For instance, the UNAIDS initiative in Côte-d'Ivoire discouraged treatment with the effective triple therapy (the cocktail of three ARVs taken together, known as highly active antiretroviral therapy or HAART) because only therapy with *two* drugs was subsidized. Two drugs are, however, only partially effective at suppressing the virus, giving it time to become resistant to an inadequate drug regimen.

I was told that this decision was made so that more patients could receive ARVs. This was a rationale that reflected the sense that getting drugs into bodies was urgent and the erroneous assumption that two out of three drugs would be two-thirds as effective as three drugs. Unfortunately, it is not. This is because a two-drug regimen only works for six months while a three-drug regimen works for many years—as many as ten or more. Even worse, treatment with only two drugs rapidly causes the virus to become resistant to the drugs, which explains why two-drug combinations don't work after six months. As a result, many of those who were treated as part of the UNAIDS initiative acquired resistance to ARV drugs, compromising their subsequent chances of successful treatment. From interviews I conducted at the time, it became clear to me that the pressure to evaluate the program in terms of "numbers treated" played a significant role. Local physicians wanted to use the drugs, and activists wanted to get them. At the same time, the implications of inadequate treatment were sidestepped by local and international authorities, who wanted results fast and were unwilling to be seen as contesting the decisions of their counterparts.

The local and global political context in which the program was deployed was, in this respect, significant. The French had for some time been arguing that treatment needed to be part of the fight against AIDS in developing countries. Côte-d'Ivoire, the jewel in the postcolonial French crown, was to be a showcase. Similarly, UNAIDS was being held accountable to a constituency of AIDS activists increasingly vocal about the issue of access to antiretroviral drugs in developing countries. At one level, then, the UNAIDS Ivoirian initiative was more about showing that something was being done for political ends both domestically and internationally than about achieving meaningful public health results. It was the very power of antiretrovirals to save lives that meant that results could be measured in these quantitative terms.

When I argued, on biological grounds, that it would make more sense to treat the same number of people with triple therapy for a shorter period of time to save money, people told me that this would be politically difficult, as no one wanted to be seen as stopping treatment—a reasonable enough argument from the political perspective.[9] The choice to ration drugs in this way was therefore the result of a murky tangle of institutional micropolitics—the tactical struggles over power and drugs, involving local and international officials, activists, and patients. This tangle is described in great detail in a remarkable evaluation of the program that, it must be stressed, benefited from an unprecedented degree of cooperation from Ivoirian officials. The Ivoirian government's transparency and willingness to be held to account by both its own populations and the international community contrasts with the relative opacity surrounding the international actors that were also part of the program (Msellati, Vidal, and Moatti 2001).

As a result, the biological fates of those who participated in the program were altered, with consequences still to be determined. If no further treatment programs had come about, even this partial therapy may have extended many lives, but not by much. Those who had received only two drugs had taken an inadequate treatment that led to their HIV's becoming resistant to their ARVs, and often to other ARV drugs. That made it more difficult to treat these patients with the drugs that became more available after 2002 since resistance meant many of the drugs could no longer work. Those who remained "naïve," or never got the drugs, actually had better odds of responding to the newer therapies.[10] The triage enacted by the UNAIDS pilot program occurred on a much larger scale than the informal mechanisms experimented with by early HIV groups. Triage created biological differences between those who received full treatment, inadequate treatment (which limited options for successful long-term therapy), and no treatment.

Moreover, a large number of the initial group of patients were found to already harbor a drug-resistant virus—certain evidence that they had already had partial access to ARVs before the initiative (Adjé, Cheingsong, Roels, Maurice, Djomand, Verbiest, Hertogs et al. 2001). This important observation has been repeated in other African countries (see Nkengasong, Adjé-Touré and Weidle 2004, 9) and indicates that even without structured treatment programs, some patients in some places do gain partial access to treatment, resulting in suboptimal treatment and increasing chances of viral resistance to the drugs. Treatment programs, however they ration drugs, are thus confronting the biological effects of earlier triage.

Emergence of Global Treatment Activism

In America and Europe, an important goal of AIDS activism was to obtain treatment for the disease by lobbying for research and speeding up the regulatory process in order to get "drugs into bodies." The result was a blending of activism, clinical research, and medical practice (S. Epstein 1996). Consequently, drug approval and distribution were fast-tracked. Over a decade after the advent of this biomedical activism in the North, the year 2000 marked a watershed in the global fight against AIDS and, arguably, in the broader issue of globalization and public health. The therapeutic revolution heralded by combination antiretroviral therapy catalyzed consciousness of the implications of global health inequities.

When awareness crystallized in 1996 that the drug cocktails were going to let people with HIV live, treating people with HIV in developing countries was almost unthinkable—the cocktails cost upward of fifteen thousand dollars annually, required complex monitoring, and were clearly out of reach for poor countries with health budgets that amounted to no more than a few dollars per person. The issue began to surface in 1998, as symbolized by that year's World AIDS Conference's slogan: "Bridging the gap," a timid acknowledgment that "one world one hope," the slogan of the 1996 Vancouver conference, was certainly not the case. The decision to hold the 2000 conference in Durban, South Africa—the first time this conference had been held outside of a Northern country—catalyzed activists and media interest. Simultaneously, South African president Thabo Mbeki's public skepticism about whether HIV "caused" AIDS precipitated a media storm that focused attention on the catastrophic dimensions of the epidemic in Africa in general, and in South Africa in particular.

The result was unprecedented attention to the issue of access to HIV treatments and, increasingly, the state of public health in Africa and indeed throughout the developing world in the age of globalization. This visibility was largely due to the efforts of a transnational coalition of health and AIDS activist NGOs that had taken up the issue of access to HIV treatment in developing countries. This issue resonated with broader concerns—and coalitions—that sprang up around a number of issues posed by globalization, in effect making access to treatment—and the global intellectual property laws thought to impede this—a signature issue for the antiglobalization movement.

Spearheaded by a professional and effective campaign led by Médecins sans frontières, Health Action International, and the Consumer Project on Technology, public and political attention focused on the prohibitive cost of these drugs (Stolberg 2001). These NGOs had been active advocates for equity in access to health for many years but had gained little support for the issue in international policy circles or with the general public. The lack of access to AIDS medicines gave them a high-profile issue and, most importantly, political traction. Although AIDS activist groups in the North quickly rallied to the campaign, it is unclear why they did not join the bandwagon until a full five years after the therapeutic revolution took place. In 1998 ACT-UP Paris drew attention to the issue at the AIDS Conference in Geneva, but unfortunately, in this case the group's lack of professionalism and their inability to back up rhetoric with solid policy undermined their credibility.

The increasingly professionalized NGOs of the AIDS industry and multilateral organizations such as UNAIDS and WHO belatedly joined the call for greater access to treatment. This was a staggering shift for some organizations, which had historically been supportive of the international consensus on the protection of intellectual property and had consistently backed away from any measures that might threaten pharmaceutical industry profits (Peschard 2001). Claiming the mantle of treatment activism occasionally led to jarring scenes. Spokespeople who had vehemently argued against treatment for people with HIV were just as vehemently arguing the opposite a few months later. Privately, the emphasis on treatment worried the more established NGOs. They believed that treatment was too expensive and would take away money from prevention efforts—an understandable concern to the extent that they believed they were competing for money from a fixed AIDS "pot." People I spoke to who worked for multilateral organizations echoed these concerns.

As a result of the access-to-treatment campaign and the media attention it drew, through 2000 and 2001 a succession of declarations announced dramatic price reductions in the cost of these drugs. Drug prices collapsed once the Indian generic pharmaceuticals manufacturer, CIPLA, offered to make the nine antiretrovirals it produces in India available at cost to African countries. Subsequent price cuts by "big pharma," as the research and development (R&D) pharmaceutical industry that makes patented drugs is called, followed. In early 2008, GlaxoSmithKline, the world's largest pharmaceuticals firm, announced even further price cuts for drugs to the developing world.

Therapeutic Citizenship

I have elaborated on the notion of therapeutic citizenship in this chapter to show how patients' sense that they were contributing to developing treatments for others motivated participation in the first clinical trials in the North, which led to the discovery of effective therapy. In Burkina Faso and Côte-d'Ivoire, clinical trials were a way of accessing some form of care where it was otherwise nonexistent. Clinical trials, in a sense, produced a population of people who knew they were HIV positive, even as the trials themselves included only a few and excluded many. This injustice triggered an initial AIDS activism that led many to join or set up groups of people living with HIV. Gradually, a trickle of supplies of the life-saving drugs was obtained by therapeutic pioneers like Abdoulaye, who used their contacts and their skills to make the necessary connections and set up the drug pipelines. These were years of triage, where painful decisions had to be made as to who would get the drugs and live, and who would not and as a result eventually die. It became clear that what was at stake was life itself. Triage was initially conducted on a micro scale, within small groups, before expanding to a broader level as pilot programs ramped up supplies that were, nevertheless, insufficient to meet demand. What emerged out of this experience was a powerful sense of rights—to treatment and, in effect, to life—and of responsibilities to others. That sense of responsibility was heightened by the experience of having lived through those early years of drug rationing and the profound conviction that no other person should die for want of drugs. These profoundly ethical predicaments shaped the therapeutic citizenship that emerged in places where other forms of citizenship could not be relied upon to secure life itself.

This therapeutic citizenship contrasts with other forms of "biological citizenship" that are also mediated by biomedical categories (Petryna 2002, Rose and Novas 2004). These authors use the term "biological citizenship" to index the way in which biomedical science and categories are used to categorize and manage individuals and adjudicate their claims for compensation; it also refers to how individuals act on their lives through biomedicine. Central to these notions of biological citizenship has been an understanding of the role of the state and other large, stable institutions as guarantors of health care and social security. Therapeutic citizenship is also conditioned by biological knowledge and biomedical practice. It differs from the "biological citizenship" described by Rose and Novas and Petryna in that it arises where large, stable institutions that can grant access to life-saving therapy are absent. It is a thin citizenship, solely focused on a particular disease. Since it is active in a setting where the disease may be the only way to get any of the material security one usually associates with citizenship, it takes on a particular poignancy."

Triage

Life-saving antiretroviral treatments arrived against a background of crushing poverty. Efforts to organize communities with HIV had put into place technologies used to foster self-help and elicit testimonials. With the arrival of ARVs, these practices were used for selecting those who would receive the treatments and those who would not. This is what I call "triage." Triage is an operation that differentiates people into groups based on specific criteria, such as those who require immediate medical attention from those who do not. We have seen how biomedical criteria occluded subtle forms of evaluating differences and selected people based on their perceived value to organizations, communities, or programs. The prioritizing of those who should be rescued and the forms of value they constituted resulted from dire material circumstances. The pragmatic assemblage of procedures and technologies not intended for this purpose was the rational response to these circumstances. This was life-boat ethics. Life itself was at stake. Tentative forms of solidarity and social relations, anchored by the biomedical predicament of being infected with HIV and shared through testimonials and confessional narratives, gave way to competition and an emerging therapeutic citizenship. Triage thus linked procedures for selecting people, the ways in which people seek to transform themselves, practices of "telling" the truth about the self, and the paradoxical affirmation of citizenship.

The politics of triage are not seamless. They occur at multiple levels: within groups and in practices that, despite the intentions behind their use, selected those that would receive treatment; between international agencies and governments; in policies that used selection criteria to ration treatment in the global arena; and in the political and economic structures that produce and enforce the global inequalities decried by global treatment activists. These are politics that are linked to social and biological practices of self-transformation; the former through narrative and experiential technologies of the self, the latter through pharmaceuticals. What unites them is a central concern with life itself. This concern institutes practices of triage in procedures that explicitly or implicitly separate those who will receive life-giving treatment from those who will not. It is a politics that has leveraged some meaningful political changes; but it remains, for the most part, turned toward the predicament of individual survival.

The notion of citizenship highlights the political dimensions of the patterns of resort that brought people diagnosed with HIV to self-help groups and the social relations that resulted. These trajectories were attempts to influence fate, to enroll others in one's destiny, and to shape how the future played out in the organization of communities around HIV. They recall Harris's prophetic movement and the voluntary associations during colonial times. The historical unfolding of Harris's prophetic movement and colonial voluntary associations revealed the potential for new technologies to unleash political energies.

Can the emergence of therapeutic citizenship and triage be attributed to the peculiarities of the local character or were they imposed from the outside? Are they historical aberrations that will wither away as mass treatment programs are deployed to address the crisis? Moreover, what are the implications of the introduction of these novel mechanisms that sort people out based on their need for treatment? The next three chapters will answer these questions by unearthing the historical substructure of triage and its consequences, examining selection, rationing, and truth telling, respectively.

BIOPOWER
············

Fevers, Tribes, and Bulldozers

In 1999 a colleague and I were arguing about how to improve the way we treated and followed patients at the Abidjan AIDS clinic where we both worked. I had been trying to conduct an epidemiological study and had realized that some patients had been doubly entered into the database under slightly different names, making it impossible to know exactly how many patients we were treating. As a result, we were trying to devise a system of "coding" patients so that each patient would have a unique identifier, the equivalent of a Medicare or social insurance number. My colleague insisted that we devise a system involving patients' initials and date of birth. It seemed a sensible enough idea but proved unworkable once it became clear that not only did many patients have very similar names but that name and date of birth varied according to which piece of ID they used. As was the case in many developing countries in colonial times and even later, parents often obtained a birth certificate only when they needed it—most often, once they had decided that a child should go to school. The expense of school fees meant that parents would often choose to wait until a child was seven- or eight-years-old and had demonstrated the ability to succeed academically. As a result, the birth date was often brought forward to make the child appear younger, so as not to compromise the child's chances of advancing through the educational system, as age cut-offs are used to select out older and, it is assumed, less gifted children.[1] In other cases, individuals obtained birth certificates or identity cards later in life, with birth date and even name adjusted to best suit their purposes.

What became clear in the course of our attempt to improve the clinic's patient care was that there was no reliable way to "fix" the identity of patients precisely; because the state did not do so, it was not the guarantor of identity. (Think of the cases of mistaken identity on U.S. "no-fly" lists.) We ended up devising a system where the clinic took on this role by assigning a unique identifier based on the sequence in which the patients registered—in effect, supplanting one of the fundamental roles of the state solely for the task of managing therapy. Indeed, as programs have now scaled up throughout Africa, they have been confronted with a similar dilemma. All must use some kind of technology of identification—in some places, smart cards are even used—to correctly identify beneficiaries of treatment.

We decided to issue patients ID cards with their unique identification numbers, which would allow a reliable method of tracking them independently of any other documents they might have. I began to realize that for many patients this was the most meaningful symbol of citizenship they had. For most of them, the state existed only as absence or unfulfilled promise. Many of the state's basic functions in providing for the welfare of its citizens were instead assured by the social relations that were cobbled together in lieu of the state, such as family, but also groups such as Light for AIDS and Positive Nation. The international agencies, NGOs, and humanitarian clinics that stepped in to provide basic services for HIV functioned as a double of the state. Being HIV positive, in this context, constituted a kind of parallel and derivative citizenship. Clinic ID cards provided access to treatment and health—life itself.

Foucault (1978, 135–37) coined the term "biopower" to refer to the modern European state's growing preoccupation with marshaling the vital forces of its population in the nineteenth century through the exercise of power over life. Accordingly, biopower refers to a continuum between, at one end, a battery of measures aimed at improving population health through urban sanitation, economic policy, and public health efforts and, at the other end, interventions aimed at individuals that sought to discipline, regulate, and monitor bodily conduct. The "government of the living" thus linked two poles: a "biopolitics of population" and an "anatomo-politics" of individual bodies. The premodern, monarchical state was not concerned with governing the lives of its citizens in intimate detail. It exercised sovereignty by waging war, enforcing borders, collecting taxes, and excluding or even eliminating threatening elements. With the modern state, biopower emerges as key to the exercise of sovereignty.

Recall how epidemiological "maps" of the population informed efforts to respond to the AIDS epidemic: these were the seroprevalence figures that preoccupied Madame Janvier and Abdoulaye. The response deployed a battery of tools that increasingly sought to identify and manage HIV-positive individuals. Prevention efforts were intensified as confessional technologies were used to elicit testimonials. Yet as treatment became available, these technologies in effect, and largely unintentionally, triaged who would be treated. These efforts can be viewed as a rudimentary form of biopower. It is a selective form of biopower because it focuses on a single issue—HIV—to the exclusion of others. Moreover these efforts concentrated on specific populations—people living with HIV and those at "high risk" such as sex workers and youth—that it sought to call into being and manage in order to control the epidemic in the entire population. Epidemiology and mass campaigns were linked to confessional technologies, conjugating a biopolitics of population and an anatomo-politics of individual bodies.

Foucault traced the rise of biopower through a historical examination of the rise of the modern European state. In Burkina Faso and Côte-d'Ivoire, NGOs and self-help groups mobilized the biopolitical technologies deployed to combat HIV. This points to a curious, "nongovernmental" biopower that disseminates through a patchwork of international organizations and community groups. What might be the consequences of this selective and partial exercise of biopower? What, exactly, is at stake?

To explore these questions, this chapter will examine how biopower was consolidated in colonial French West Africa. Following colonial conquest, the rise of a microbial approach to controlling epidemics made it possible for biomedical technologies to target the bodies of Africans despite racist notions of biological difference. Administrative technologies were used to classify and group populations, in the process solidifying "ethnicity" into a substrate for governmental practice. Finally, urban planning materialized a differential calculus of the value of citizens that erased local notions of kinship. This nonetheless shaped urban life and the forms of tactical citizenship that resulted. Before the time of AIDS, France exercised sovereignty through processes that differentiated people, selected them, and calculated their value. These key biopolitical practices and the struggles they shaped constituted colonial sovereignty as they in effect "made up" people and fashioned citizenship outside and even against the colonial state. This historical exploration illuminates how a newer, nongovernmental biopower could take root.

Contemporary efforts to respond to the HIV epidemic that map populations according to their seroprevalence rates, screen them to identify "cases," and organize them into groups in order to "empower" and eventually treat them, parallel colonial biopower. That triage played out in these contemporary efforts testifies to the lingering effects of earlier procedures for differentiating, grouping, and directing populations. It also suggests that the struggles that shape biopower in the time of AIDS may in fact constitute an elementary form of sovereignty: a power over life and death. This is a partial and selective sovereignty that emerges in struggles over who gets treated.

I begin this story by focusing on the systematic practices used to sort and group people in Côte-d'Ivoire in the time before AIDS. This is not a history of social difference. Rather, my approach here is *genealogical*. It uncovers historical phenomena that, in light of the present, can be seen as ancestral forms onto which technologies of the self and triage could graft. This chapter begins with the colonial era because it introduced the systematic classification of larger territorial populations in order to make distinctions *across* groups. This occurred when, after successfully waging a war of conquest, France found itself confronted with the problem of asserting its sovereignty over a potentially hostile population it knew little about. That problem was intensified in the colonial capital, the seat of colonial government that was both a relay for exercising colonial domination and a hub for massive migratory flows that concentrated colonial populations in one place.

Sovereignty

France formally claimed sovereignty over the West African territory known as Côte-d'Ivoire in 1893, aiming to bolster its presence along the West African coasts in the face of British competition (Atger 1962). Its capital was located in Grand-Bassam, one of the original fortified trading posts with a large French trading community. Bassam, located at the confluence of the Comoé River and the Ébrié Lagoon, offered a natural hub for connecting commerce in the interior with sea-going vessels. When it became the capital of the new colony, only a narrow strip of land along the ocean was effectively under French control; the remaining territory existed merely as an empty space on maps. In order to assert sovereignty over the unmapped territory, France followed a policy of "peaceful penetration," attempting to conquer the interior through a series of missions empowered to negotiate the imposition of French rule. Peaceful penetration was a failure, punctuated by armed revolts requiring muscular French intervention. In 1908 the territory of the colony was still not under French control. This led France to implement a vigorous policy of "pacification" that was in effect a war of occupation waged through the destruction of resistant villages, the massacre of able-bodied men, and the taking of hostages to win over recalcitrant chiefs. Overall it was "one of the most enduring and most brutally repressed resistance struggles in West African history" (Weiskel 1980, xvii). Transformed into a theater of combat, the empty space on the map of the interior was brought under French control by 1915 after significant bloodshed (Coquery-Vidrovitch 1992, 291–98).

Grand-Bassam was spared bloodshed; nonetheless, its days as the capital were numbered. It turned out to be a less-than-ideal port. Added to this inconvenience, a rather more dramatic problem emerged, as epidemics of yellow fever succeeded each other at the close of the nineteenth century. These epidemics were legion throughout the French *comptoirs* (trading posts) of the West African coast in the nineteenth century. They decimated the European populations who lived there and took on added political significance with the establishment of a permanent administrative colony. Bassam's yellow fever epidemics occurred in 1899, 1902, and 1903,[2] the last one killing nearly all of Bassam's European inhabitants.[3] The later outbreaks led to near panic among the settlers, and a mounting rhetoric of epidemiological catastrophe produced by colonial administrators finally convinced metropolitan authorities that the administrative capital would have to be moved.[4] The village of Adjamé, twenty-five kilometers further east on the lagoon, was finally settled in 1899. Renamed Bingerville after the colony's founder and first governor, the site was considered particularly clement, as it was situated on a plateau one hundred meters above sea level and swept by breezes, thus less prone to malaria (Wondji 1976). While Bingerville was to become the administrative capital, another site with a harbor was chosen for the colony's economic capital: Abidjan. French conquest conjured up a local capital from which rule could be exercised, and it materialized as a biopolitical fortress shaped by a double threat: a potentially rebellious population and tropical disease (Suret-Canale 1982; Wondji 1982).

Fevers

For Europeans in the nineteenth century, Africa was reputed to be "the white man's grave," a metaphor whose origin has been traced to the seventeenth-century experience of the British in Sierra Leone. The tropical fevers that decimated Europeans were attributed to toxic air, "malaria," reflecting the prevailing miasma theory of disease causation that attributed illness to unhealthy environments. The miasma theory has dominated Western medical thinking from the Greeks on and was dethroned only after Pasteur's demonstration of the microbial origin of disease in the late nineteenth century (Arnold 1996). In Africa, miasma theory and other environmentalist ideas of disease causation persisted even as the discoveries of Pasteur lead to widespread acceptance of the germ theory in the metropole. This profoundly structured the way in which Europeans sought to preserve their health.

That Côte-d'Ivoire was rife with tropical fevers confirmed suspicions, in the colonial mind, that the languid climate festered with pathology. This fed a lurid array of representations and practices obsessed with both the environment and racial difference. Africans were assumed to be "acclimatized" to the noxious environments that bred disease—an assumption that confirmed prevailing ideas of racial difference as biological and conveniently absolved colonial authorities of any responsibility for their health. Reflecting both the colonial logic of bioracial difference and the imperative of protecting settler health, Abidjan was divided into two zones. One, higher up and healthfully breezy, with European architecture and amenities, was intended for settlers. To this day it is called the Plateau, like other European quarters in many French colonial cities all over the world. Lower down around the dank lagoon were the townships reserved for Africans. Miasma theory gave credence to these policies of racial segregation, which were enacted throughout the colonial world. Swanson (1977) dubbed the application of these segregationist ideologies to colonial urban planning the "sanitation syndrome."[5]

As result of this racist sanitation policy, in the prewar period, the majority of Africans in Abidjan were consigned to live outside the borders of the airy European city, crowded into impromptu housing. In the indigenous quarter of Cocody, Africans lived in "lamentable shacks, huts built of dried mud, bits of crates and old petrol canisters" which, a colonial commentator reported, "make Cocody the most insalubrious agglomeration."[6] Colonial anxieties about native hygiene, prevalent in the 1910s and 1920s, were heightened by the memory of the epidemics that had ravaged Grand-Bassam and led to the establishment of Abidjan, and were expressed in a series of reports, ordinances, and recommendations that enacted an imaginary *cordon sanitaire* (hygienic border) around the European quarter by displacing Africans from the Plateau. The cruel irony was that segregationist policies, by concentrating poor populations in unhealthy conditions, worked to spread infectious disease—a self-fulfilling prophecy that provided fertile ground for epidemics and, subsequently, campaigns to eradicate them.

Decline of Miasma Theory

The discovery in the early 1900s that malaria was caused by mosquito-borne plasmodium parasites marked an important shift by which African and European bodies were now taken to be biologically commensurable. The biological condition of African bodies—as potential carriers of disease—therefore became relevant to colonial attempts to protect settler health. Advances in biomedical science thus substituted the idea of the "dirty savage" for that of the "diseased native" (Packard 1989). They indicated that disease eradication would require more than segregating "natives"; it would require that they be targeted for biomedical intervention.

In the years between the two world wars, prevailing ideas of Africans as biologically different from Europeans faded away. In their place emerged a theory of microbial disease causation that powerfully demonstrated that human biology was a workably universal standard for addressing epidemics. This theory was borne by a cadre of young physicians and scientists who were then known as "Pasteurians." This movement followed Pasteur, who was the father of the microbe theory of disease. Pasteur's experiments and rhetoric were convincing enough to influence French state policy. Pasteurian interventions—such as vaccination—demonstrated success once they had mobilized the state resources they needed for implementation. The French medical corps, bidden to miasma theories, was slow to come about to the new ideas and resisted acknowledging the role of microbes until the very end of the nineteenth century. Although the official vector of Pasteurianism, the Société de Pathologie Exotique, was founded in 1907, it took another twenty years for public health measures based on Pasteurian ideas to be adopted in the colonies.[7]

In addition to the usefulness of miasma theory for legitimating segregationist measures, other factors delayed acceptance of Pasteurian ideas in colo-

rcsm too few physcns

no infln GWW1

nial French Africa. Colonial physicians were few and far between, having to cover large territories, which obliged them to be frequently absent as they often had to travel long distances to minister to ill settlers. Despite the creation of a Native Health Service (Assistance médicale indigène) in 1905, these army physicians were spread too thinly to have much of an effect on native health. When they weren't traveling, their time was largely spent dealing with local administrative problems. These took priority over catching up with the new, Pasteurian ideas. Colonial laissez-faire, coupled with fear that a too-accurate portrait of health problems would scare off future settlers and investors, conspired to keep health records and statistics patchy and masked the morbidity and mortality due to infectious diseases in the population. The First World War interrupted whatever institutional continuity existed within the colonial public health service, at a time when the continent was devastated by the great influenza pandemic of 1919 and concurrent epidemics of river blindness, sleeping sickness, and leprosy, triggered by the migratory movements inherent to the new colonial economy. As a result, there was little institutional infrastructure for conveying Pasteurian theories. And finally, the corps of African health assistants was poorly trained, often overwhelmed with adapting to the odd routines of the white man's medicine, and thus was unlikely to serve as a conduit for even newer and stranger ideas (Bado 1996, 151–90). The resistance to Pasteurian ideas constituted an opposition to what they implied: that all races were biologically equivalent. Once this resistance was overcome, colonial anxieties about epidemics and Africans could be addressed within a single, unified approach.

Pasteurization

The crystallization of Pasteurianism in a network of tropical Pasteur Institutes, French military medical academies, and a reinvigorated colonial public health administration slowly began to overcome these barriers in the 1920s. The tropical Pasteur Institutes were founded in the late nineteenth century throughout the French empire, most notably in Saigon and Nha-Trang (both in Indochina) and Tunis (Moulin 1992). The institutes pursued research, applying Pasteurian ideas to tropical illnesses. Meanwhile, Pasteurian ideas were transmitted through the military medical schools of Bordeaux and Lyon, which trained future colonial medics.

Preoccupation with the biological condition of African populations grew after the First World War, when France found itself with a demographic defi-

cit caused by the deaths of so many young men and compounded by the decrease in fertility that followed. France's African colonies were worse off than
France, having been devastated by epidemics of flu, plague, and trypanosomiasis (commonly known as sleeping sickness). The effect of these epidemics
was exacerbated by the precarious nutritional status of the population, as
colonial forced-labor practices took men away from subsistence farming. In-
fertility—the product of declining nutrition and sexually transmitted diseases
introduced by Europeans—registered at epidemic levels. The decline of the
African population throughout the colonies spurred a metropolitan near-
hysteria about the imminent "extinction of the Black race," a worrisome prospect given the colonial economy's reliance on African labor and the hopes it
embodied for France's postwar economic recovery. A decrease in the labor
pool available to the colonies would have seriously compromised the economic viability of the colonies in which France had considerable stakes.

The Pasteurians' commitment to the vector theory of disease reshaped
colonial public health policy from the 1930s onward, in the form of campaigns
against endemic infectious diseases that were developed in response to concerns about African depopulation.[8] The success of the campaigns fueled the
rise of Pasteurianism, generating powerful evidence in support of microbial
theory and the implication that all humans (whatever their race) were biologically equivalent. An unintended boost to the Pasteurians was the establishment of the only medical school for Africans in Dakar, partly to remedy the
deficiencies of colonial physicians' African assistants. The school opened in
1918, and in 1920 its mission was described as being to "clean up the country,
instruct the Native, give him essential notions of Hygiene, protect him from
preventable illnesses, and fortify the race to increase its capacity for work and
wealth" (quoted in Bado 1996, 217). By the mid-1920s, Pasteurian ideas had
achieved medical acceptance and institutionalization, and the new colonial
school of medicine assured a wider audience and the diffusion of Pasteur's
revolution through a trained class of African intermediaries.

At first, Pasteurians' influence remained confined to the realm of colonial public health campaigns aimed at eradicating endemic tropical infectious diseases. These mobile campaigns scoured the countryside of the French
colonies, largely leaving cities untouched. Pasteurianism, with its strategy of
geometrically dividing up the territory with a tactical public health apparatus, was easier to implement in rural areas, where sleeping sickness and leprosy eradication campaigns were among Africans' most feared experiences

of colonialism. In the 1920s and 1930s, mobile teams scoured the countryside screening for trypanosomiasis by lining up villagers and palpating their cervical lymph nodes. Those with swollen nodes had their lymph fluid sampled with a needle aspirate. People found to have the parasite were subjected to painful and, it turned out, ineffective injections. As a result, during this period villagers often fled into the bush when word spread that public health teams were in the vicinity. Some Ivoirians even had their cervical lymph nodes excised by charlatan surgeons to avoid the injections, demonstrating how, at times, colonial public health measures generated radical forms of resistance to biomedicine.[9] Nonetheless, the success of Pasteurian biomedicine to control epidemics set the stage for subsequent campaigns to address infectious diseases.

Biomedicine and the Value of African Labor

In the city, once microbes replaced racial difference as an explanation for tropical disease, Africans were seen as potential harbors of dangerous pathogens. Culture replaced biological difference as an explanation for the peril Africans represented to European health and became the target of a broad array of measures that sought to contain this threat through surveillance and the imposition of "hygienic" practices to Africans' ways of life. The realization that African labor was needed to produce wealth for France produced an important shift in these early public health policies, which initially only sought to protect settlers from the imagined threat Africans posed to their health. As the minister of colonies famously told his officials in the colonies, it was now time to adopt policies that would *"faire du nègre"* (literally "breed Negroes"). As a result, colonial authorities were successfully lobbied in the early twenties to undertake measures to "save the Black race." Africans now became the target of pronatalist policies that sought to increase "quantity," while worker health programs focused on "quality" (Echenberg 1994).

Biomedicine became the preferred approach to managing the African population, its efficacy anchored in the recognition that despite racial "difference," Africans shared a common biology with Europeans. In French West Africa (known by the French acronym for Afrique occidentale française, AOF), the number of physicians increased, from around 30 at the outbreak of the First World War, to 92 in 1925, and 133 in 1926. The health budget almost tripled from 1925 to 1927; every colony was instructed to devote between 7 and 12 percent of its budget to health (Bado 1996, 228). Timid investments were made in the creation of a public health system organized around central hospitals with diagnostic facilities, peripheral dispensaries that would assist hospitals in ascertaining and monitoring the diseases that afflicted the population, and mobile campaigns to stamp out preventable diseases. These early investments disproportionately favored cities and towns, shifting the clinical gaze of colonial power from the rural areas—and the epidemic eradications campaigns conducted there—to the city. This established a pattern that was reinforced when more substantial investments were made after the Second World War.

In summary, the rise of a colonial public health apparatus was thus made possible by the emergence of Africans as biological subjects in their own right, as Pasteurian theories and practices swept the colonies. As African labor became increasingly important to producing wealth for France, the colonial preoccupation with African health grew. Formerly repressive measures aimed at segregating Africans and Europeans gave way to the deployment of measures focused on producing healthy African workers, including the development of a rudimentary biomedical infrastructure. Crude practices of bioracial differentiation that sacrificed the health of Africans in the mistaken belief that this would shield settlers from tropical diseases gave way to practices that valued the health of African workers. A regime of valuing settler life to the exclusion of others gave way to one that tentatively deployed a set of mechanisms that preserved the hierarchy of value that placed the European on top. As the eclipse of a crude, bioracist triage ushered in a biomedical approach to managing the population, health and labor acquired commensurable forms of value. This regime of value enabled subtle forms of triage that mapped new social categories in the colonial economy.

Ethnographic Sorting

In response to the threat tropical disease posed to colonial rule, the Pasteurian demonstration that African bodies, as biological entities, could be targeted for intervention with impressive results was an important step in focusing colonial power on the problem of "life." Colonial concern with the biological lives of Africans was paralleled by the desire to "map" the population using administrative technologies for classifying humans. This began once the territory was conquered, as exploratory missions constituted a systematic program that linked mapping the territory with naming the populations that inhabited it. The colonial state conjugated a cartographic project with an ethnographic one (Chauveau and Dozon 1987). Mapping was both an instrument of rule, construed as a rationalized relationship between the state and its territory, and a practice that constituted that rule (Biggs 1999). The project was a belabored one: the colonial presence required vigorous military support, and colonial administrators were few and far between, did not speak local languages, and, in the beginning, had few local people they could rely on to help them carry out their administrative duties (W. Cohen 1971).[10]

The task of mapping the colony and its inhabitants built on the work of the French ethnographer-explorer Maurice Delafosse, whose linguistic ethnography in 1904 formed the basis for a "genealogy of races" of the territory. This ethnic inventory of the colony, while viewed as provisory and incomplete even by its author, congealed quickly and changed little thereafter. The colonial state did not require further details to govern and contented itself with grouping tribes into "families" such as the Kru or the Akan. Naming was part and parcel of the "cartographic reason" of the state, which used tribal families to divide the territory into large swaths—the "Senoufo country" or "Baoulé country"—made up of smaller tribal zones. Solidification of ethnic categories was not just a product of mechanical ascription by the state; by the 1920s, "natives" themselves were appropriating these labels in their dealings with colonial authorities.[11]

Implementing metropolitan policies aimed at economic development in the 1930s, the colonial state began to invest heavily in the development of a plantation economy. Correspondingly, it shifted from a cartographic approach to the "natives" to an ethnographic one, differentiating ethnicities according to imagined aptitudes and predispositions. Mapping gave way to culturalizing. Terms such as "quarrelsome," "unstable," or "admirable" were used to classify groups in order to better manage their role in the colonial economy. This labeling was also a self-fulfilling prophecy characterized by "working misunderstandings," processes of misrecognition that nonetheless established the framework that would govern relations between "natives," the state, and the colonial economy.[12] By sorting out people through the attribution of ethnic identities, the colonial state made ethnicity into a powerful technology for reading and producing social difference. New social groups, such as the Baoulé, materialized.

Census information has consistently identified, from colonial times to the present, the Baoulé as the largest ethnic group in Abidjan and Côte-d'Ivoire. Not insignificantly, the founding president of the First Republic, Félix Houphouët-Boigny, was Baoulé, as was his successor, Henri Konan Bédié. In contemporary Côte-d'Ivoire, the Baoulé are considered the politically dominant ethnicity in this most multicultural nation. The demographic history of the Baoulé, however, contains a puzzle: the depression of the 1930s, like the demographic crisis immediately after the First World War, shrank the population of the colony in the face of widespread food shortages. Yet from 1936 to 1948, according to census information and colonial records, when the rest of the colony was just barely recovering from the demographic effects of the crisis and starting to stabilize population loss, the Baoulé population actually *grew* at an astonishing rate of 4.8 percent per year, far above what was considered the natural demographic growth rate of 2 percent. However, the Baoulé population shrank by 4.4 percent from 1948 to 1950, but then spurted again at an astonishing 8.5 percent while the colony's aggregate population was growing at only 4.6 percent (Chauveau 1987). How did this happen?

In fact, colonial rule "made" the Baoulé into the dominant ethnicity. This assertion is supported by the inability of rival hypotheses to explain the growth in Baoulé numbers. One such rival hypothesis is the political explanation that claims that demographic dominance leads to political dominance, which in turn leads to individuals "converting" to the politically dominant ethnicity for pragmatic reasons, swelling its demographic ranks. In contrast to this "snowball" hypothesis, culturalist explanations have looked to marriage patterns and kinship structures to explain demographic increases. Baoulé kinship structure is matrilineal (meaning that children "belong" to the mother's brother rather than their father) and polygamous (men may have more than one wife). Exogamy was widely accepted, and offspring were recognized as Baoulé. The low rate of endogenous polygamy (that is, marriage among Baoulé), it was argued, freed up Baoulé women for exogamy. However, neither explanation is convincing. The Baoulé were never demographically dominant *anywhere* other than in central Côte-d'Ivoire until 1955, when they became the dominant ethnic group in Abidjan. Political dominance did not occur until Houphouët solidified his hold over the state and the party after independence in 1961—and *after* both demographic spurts. Finally, the Baoulé were not the only matrilineal society in Ivoirian space. In fact, the coastal population was largely Akan and matrilineal, like the Baoulé, but it did not experience the same population growth. Political and cultural factors may have played a part, but cannot fully explain the phenomenon.

How did the colonial state then "make up" the Baoulé as a dominant ethnicity? Ethnographers and historians have observed that the Baoulé never "crystallized" a social structure. According to early informants, the term "baoulé" actually refers to a form of sacrifice performed by a group of dissidents as they left what is now Ghana in the mid-eighteenth century in a dispute over the succession to the Ashanti throne. Some of them settled in the central region of the colony, in an area that was a hub for commerce, and once there, integrated with other local groups. Flexible political and social organization allowed them to mesh with other groups, leading them to be described as an "interstitial" ethnicity (Chauveau 1987). Given the heterogeneity of Baoulé social structure, it is unlikely that they ever were a "tribe" in the sense of classical anthropology. Rather, the Baoulé were a diverse group of people who had migrated to the same geographical area, some but not all sharing the same myth of origin.

When the French conquered central Côte-d'Ivoire, they designated all inhabitants of this area as "Baoulé," conflating toponymy with ethnonymy. Here, the cartographic state relied on partial ethnographic theories to label the entire region and all the people who happened to live there as Baoulé. In this sense, the Baoulé formed a residual category, whose ranks were swelled through colonial ascription of this ethnic name to other inhabitants of a region that was already a crossroads, and therefore for whose inhabitants mobility was a way of life. In other words, mobile social groups *without* a strong cultural identity were more likely to be labeled Baoulé by the colonial state. Coupled with the tendency for exogamy shared by those the state labeled Baoulé, mobility facilitated the diffusion of the Baoulé identity. It was this process that colonial censuses registered as prodigious demographic growth. Not surprisingly, the periods of strong Baoulé demographic growth (1936 to 1948 and 1955 to 1965) coincided with the time that urbanization—and therefore mobility and outmarriage of young "Baoulé" women—was at its peak.[13]

The French distrusted those they called the Baoulé. They had fiercely resisted colonization (Weiskel 1980). As a result, the Baoulé were never assimilated into the colonial economy as a professional category, in the manner of the Dioula (as traders), the Dahomeyans (as clerks),[14] or the Agnis (as planters). The Baoulé initially entered the colonial plantation economy as laborers on plantations in the "Agni country" in southeast Côte-d'Ivoire, where colonial authorities first introduced coffee and cocoa plantations. Gradually, with accumulated savings, they purchased land from Agni and began planting for themselves. The looseness of Baoulé kinship was an asset, as planters were able to exert claims over a broader range of young male kin across lineages, compared to other groups where such claims were more tightly restricted by kinship (Hecht 1984). With urbanization, the "farming out" of young women to the towns increased Baoulé numbers, as their children adopted this identity and grew up to provide manpower on their elders' plantations, further enhancing their economic power.[15]

Ethnic labels would solidify further as they were used to distinguish immigrants (*allochtones*) from "true" "natives" (*autochtones*). This promoted the ethnicization of the economy, as specific groups followed the paths of economic differentiation they had been placed upon by French colonial policy. Groups such as the Baoulé—perhaps because of their historical experience of migration and assimilation—quickly learned the planting trade, accumulated capital, and used it to purchase land in order to become planters themselves. This led to the emergence of a native planter class, understood by some scholars as a proto-bourgeoisie (S. Amin 1967), which came to dominate politics after the Second World War through the personality of its leader, Félix Houphouët-Boigny, who would become the new independent republic's first president in 1961. The case of the Baoulé is a compelling example of how practices of sorting people may not only harden social differences but may even literally bring into being new populations over time.

In colonial Côte-d'Ivoire, ethnography was part of the science of government. It relied on practices used to name, map, and group people, a process of sorting people that was as much a reflection of the predicament of colonial rule as of a preexisting sociological reality. Once people were named, mapped, and grouped, however, these categories took social and material form—and ethnicity, in this example, became a social and even a demographic reality, as in the case of the Baoulé. At the heart of ethnicity, then, lay the colonial state (Chauveau and Dozon 1987). However, in the efforts to combat the AIDS epidemic, the state is strangely absent. In its place, NGOs, community groups, and international organizations proliferated. Nonetheless, might practices that sort or triage people in Côte-d'Ivoire's time of AIDS and the forms of therapeutic citizenship they constituted also bring into being new populations and new divisions? And, in the absence of the state, what lies at the heart of this new biomedical ethnicity? To pursue these questions, I now examine how citizenship came to be constituted against and to some extent outside the state in Abidjan.

The Rise of Citizenship in Abidjan

In the city, housing policy was the corollary of ethnographic sorting, as it divided people based on economic assumptions about their value. Housing would become a key site of struggle from the 1920s on that would persist after independence. The foundation of the colony in 1893 was in effect an annexation of the territory, which became the property of France. The French *régime foncier* (colonial property regime) was the juridical framework through which France imposed rule on the territory it had conquered, in effect expropriating and dispossessing an entire population. Already by 1900, however, the new colonial state found itself tacitly acknowledging native land claims by recognizing their title to lands they inhabited and farmed. Under this new decree, only vacant land reverted to the state, once its vacancy had been ascertained by a three-month inquest (Manou-Savina 1985). While the war of territorial conquest had apparently been won, the colonial administration was rapidly faced with "winning the peace" in a thickly inhabited territory, where land claims constituted a pragmatic resistance to the imposition of colonial rule.

Rapid urbanization from the 1950s raised the stakes for colonial authorities.[16] The colonial state was quickly confronted with another issue: what to do about the housing that was proliferating in the new coastal city of Abidjan as the population swelled with migrants from throughout the region. Because of its importance for trade, Abidjan grew rapidly after the 1920s, becoming the metropolis of the new colony and, eventually, of all French West Africa. Figures detailing population growth indicate that this must have been a headache for colonial administrators. Not having been fortified after the kind of violent confrontations that had plagued the previous capital of Bingerville, and being a trading zone, it was more permeable to population flows than Bingerville. Wishing to avoid further conflicts over land with the native population, in 1909 the state recognized such spontaneous housing post facto, issuing permits but stipulating that the state still owned the land on which these habitations were located. This was essentially a form of freehold. Another concession was granted in 1921, when the right of freeholders to sell their habitations or to be compensated in the eventuality they were displaced by the colonial state was recognized. The colonial ordinances by which Africans gained access to the land that had been taken from them differentiated people by the assumed "value" they had added to the land they occupied. A brief strike by railway workers over housing conditions in 1938 complicated things, as it highlighted the risk that housing inequalities could trigger unrest. As a result, the potential to disrupt the colonial economy would figure in that calculation of value.

In the ten years following the 1938 strike, a succession of ordinances gradually expanded property rights for urban Africans, even as a growing pile of decrees attempted to regulate "spontaneous housing." In addition to the threat of political unrest, colonial authorities worried that precarious housing conditions might lead to workers deserting the city, causing a labor shortage. Cognizant of this precariousness, in 1951 the colonial administration established a state-owned housing corporation, the Société immobilière d'habitation de Côte-d'Ivoire (SIHCI, the Côte-d'Ivoire Housing Corporation), to build affordable housing for native workers. Although the plan was not a success because the housing that was built was unaffordable, it demonstrated the growing power of urban citizenry to drive colonial policy. Colonial Abidjan was therefore shaped by policies that sought to control the population and how it lived, as well as the practices that sought to subvert and bypass these policies. Even before citizenship emerged as a political claim articulated through the nationalist movement, a pragmatic and tactical form of "citizenship" was emerging in the city, as Africans engaged with urban policies and with new urban opportunities. The attempt to govern urban Africans by differentiating them according to the value they added to the colonial project would, like the ethnic practices of differentiation discussed above, harden social difference and bring new forms of (urban) life into being.

An Urban Calculus of Value

The first public housing in Abidjan built by SIHCI was divided into three types: cheaper collective housing for laborers, built with rooms around a common courtyard, kitchens, and toilets; smaller apartments for the intermediary class of "boys" — as domestic servants were condescendingly called — and chauffeurs, which could accommodate a small family; and more spacious apartments for African white-collar workers.[17] The design of the housing and the price were determined by an all-settler commission of the Société on the basis of European assumptions about how "Africans" lived. Believing that poorer laborers lived either alone or "traditionally" in extended families, cheaper, collective housing units were built for them. The commissioners also assumed that wealthier salaried personnel—clerks and middle managers—would be more "modern" and thus prefer to live like Europeans with their smaller families in more comfortable and expensive apartment units.

The reality was the opposite. Laborers, being poorer, lived most often in a nuclear family, as they could not afford to support other family members to live in the expensive city, while wealthier workers were able to support much larger extended families. The commission fixed the prices of the dwellings as a function of wages, putting the collective housing beyond the reach of laborers unless they banded together and grouped multiple wage earners. The only people who were able to afford the new public housing were the few salaried workers who limited their expenditures to a nuclear family. The collective units went largely unoccupied, while the apartments were rented by wealthy Africans who had not been the intended beneficiaries of the SIHCI's social housing. As a result, the SIHCI's efforts ended up benefiting the elite, whereas it had originally been intended to offer subsidized housing to a representative mix of the population.

Was the case of the SIHCI just an ill-conceived policy based on faulty or inadequate data? Presumably if housing authorities had obtained good data on households, they would have been able to adjust public housing projects accordingly. This was in fact the strategy subsequently undertaken—the first household census in Abidjan occurred in 1956 but was immediately confronted with a practical obstacle. How to define a household? The French census of 1956 considered that those who lived within a single, material residence constituted a single household—obvious enough, it seemed. But, unlike in France, in Abidjan most Africans lived in *cours communes* (communal housing), whose boundaries blurred and shifted constantly. This raised another issue: how could one elaborate consistent criteria about where one household ended and another began and that could cover the almost endless permutations of building styles and living arrangements? And, how could observers be relied upon to consistently apply these criteria? These problems were never satisfactorily solved. As a result, surveys were notoriously unreliable for tracking changes in household behavior—it was never clear whether change could be attributed to shifts in household behavior or in the composition of the household itself.

One attempted solution was to redefine a household as a family unit—that is, to count all the members of a family as one household, even if they did not live in the same house. Two surveys conducted in 1963–64, just after independence, used different methodologies. One counted people living in habitation units as households (cohabitation units); the other counted people who were related as belonging to the same household (family units). Comparing the two surveys, family units were found to be *smaller* than cohabition units, an observation that ran counter to European common sense about Africans living in large, extended kinship networks. Assuming that respondents were underreporting their kinship relations, surveyors stuck to the household method. In fact, respondents were not underreporting: most urban dwellers *did* live with people they were not related to—servants, apprentices, children of friends, and so on (Le Pape 1997, 63–64), whether they were rich or poor, and the number tended to be greater for wealthier households who were able to support more dependents and employ more servants (Gibbal 1974b, 83–85).

The evolution of housing policy showed how French assumptions about African ways of life, enacted through housing policies, sliced and diced the urban population into fragments. The attempts to generate reliable knowledge about the population to inform housing policy showed how criteria for separating people into groups (such as households or families), who could then be managed through housing policy, were unable to capture the dynamics of relatedness. These dynamics were shaped both by economic constraints and the strategies people used to respond to them and could not be reduced to static notions of kinship. The French tried to separate people out according to a colonial calculus of value in order to prioritize the needs of some before others: individuals who could best contribute to the colonial economy. Colonial subjects found new ways to band together in order to meet their own needs. These were expressed according to a calculus that was different from one that located individuals within extended kinship networks.

These conflicting assessments of who was more deserving are eerie. They are eerie because they foreshadow how, in the time of AIDS, development agencies would also sort people according to a calculus of need. Since the 1990s, those who were prioritized were people with HIV who, it was assumed, required more assistance than those without: these were the people who were "valuable" for the development agencies, but also for clinical trials. Within this group, international agencies stressed helping the most "vulnerable" (for instance, women and children). This was not the same calculus as that used by the early community groups, as we have seen. For them, those who were valuable were not the most vulnerable but those whose survival was more likely to translate into benefits for the group. Like their colonial urban predecessors, those singled out in the time of AIDS also sought to generate new forms of solidarity spanning family, community groups, and the ill to ensure survival.

Urban Calculations after Independence

The empirical quest to distinguish and map the population continued and expanded in the postcolonial period from 1961 on. Designing and implementing a modern urban plan, even when this attempted to take into account the imagined local reality of Africans, shared with earlier colonial practices of ethnographic mapping the attempt to create a legible social order.[18] Just as the social cleavages produced by colonial ethnographic practice took on a life of their own, the application of categories to differentiate the urban population continued to redraw social lines, even after independence.

The sheer scope of the massive postcolonial program of housing construction dwarfed the tentative projects of the colonial state. Nothing did more to create a modern society (Le Pape 1997). Housing was to be a key pillar of state-driven modernization. According to Alain Dubresson and Alphonse Yapi-Diahou (1988, 1085), "Supported by vigorous economic growth, the State's housing policy was conceived as a rapid path to modernization, as well as a means to assuring social stability by using housing to redistribute the fruits of national growth."

The blueprint for the postcolonial state's housing agenda was the city's first *Plan d'urbanisme* begun by Badini in 1948 and ratified in 1952; a subsequent plan (the *Plan SETAP*, named after the firm that developed it) was submitted in 1960. These were the master plans outlining the direction in which the city should grow and the scope and location of public works projects for supporting that growth. This massive program of heavy public works reflected the desire to provide the city with a Western infrastructure to attract foreign investment; perhaps not coincidentally, it was the political and bureaucratic elite, overwhelmingly concentrated in the city, who benefited first from these investments (Le Pape, Vidal, and Yapi-Diahou 1991, 1–9). The plans took into account the city's alarming growth. At that time the population was doubling every six years.[19] The plans relied on demographic projections to detail significant public investments in housing.

Housing development in the 1960s was more methodical than the SIHCI's first attempt ten years earlier. A "vast programme of socio-demographic surveys" was undertaken by a battery of agencies from 1962 to 1964 under the aegis of the Planning Ministry, which processed the data from the studies between 1964 and 1967 and drew up and published a detailed action plan and program of state investments in 1969 (Anon. 1969, 26). The surveys indicated that most Abidjanais lived with nonfamily members, and this fact was taken by the surveys' commissioners to indicate that a housing shortage had gripped the city, forcing Abidjanais to live with strangers—when it was, in fact, a normal pattern of urban existence, as noted above. Massive investment in individual housing was prescribed as a remedy. However, as Le Pape has pointed out, the surveys were internally inconsistent, with wildly different results according to which methods were used. Survey methods were simplistic. They thinned the dynamic realities of urban life and failed to capture the social world of the Abidjanais. Nonetheless, the urban planners, allied with a small army of social scientists, literally constructed a new social reality (Le Pape 1997, 65–67). Eventually, thousands of individual housing units were built, requiring those that chose to live in them to simplify cohabitation arrangements in order to adapt to the new constraints. As they did so, a differentiated form of urban segregation materialized: an infrastructure of spatial triage.

Urban Form as Triage

Two years after independence, in 1963, the state housed 10 percent of Abidjanais in six thousand units. Eight years later, in 1971, this had doubled to 20 percent of Abidjanais in twelve thousand units. By 1979, on the eve of the economic crisis, an astonishing 22 percent of Abidjanais lived in state housing. But while we associate public housing with low-income tenants, in Abidjan the situation was precisely the reverse. Middle- and upper-income families benefited from the new construction, and the proportion living in private "formal" housing shrank. Meanwhile, lower-income residents remained "piled" into the "spontaneous" housing sector, which actually grew during this period: from 51 percent in 1963 to 59 percent in 1978.[20]

Through the 1960s the "spontaneous" housing sector developed along two lines, a strategy that Philippe Haeringer (1969a, 1969b) has called one of "double or nothing." Because urban residents were fully aware of the legal precariousness of shantytown constructions and the risk of demolition, dwellings were shabbily built, often of materials recycled from the port. Over time, the construction of such "precarious" housing was quasi-industrialized: the construction-destruction process was simplified, using recycled materials (such as *bidons*, plastic jugs used for gasoline) that were easily transported, assembled (creating *bidonvilles*) and, if need be, disassembled. It took three days to put up a house (Dubresson and Yapi-Diahou 1988, 1091). This was the "nothing" option: if the shantytown was demolished, losses were minimal; either the materials had been obtained free of charge or they could be carried elsewhere to build anew.

The "double" option was exercised by urban dwellers who had neither the income to purchase a home nor the contacts to get into government housing. However, these citizens had amassed sufficient resources to invest in building self-consciously modern neighborhoods. They did so by buying land from farmers immediately outside the city. However the titles to this land were not legally recognized because, since colonial times, only the state had the right to compensate traditional land claims or expropriate cultivated land for the purposes of urbanization. Nonetheless, private surveyors were hired to lay out a street grid, and citizens built "modern" houses out of durable materials. It was a significant risk since durable building materials were expensive. These new neighborhoods grew significantly in size through the 1970s, but their legal precariousness resulted in entire tracts being bulldozed by the state, meaning enormous economic losses for those whose homes had been destroyed.[21]

In the late 1970s, under pressure from the World Bank and the United States Agency for International Development (USAID), the state withdrew from the housing sector. The bank judged the state policy as noncompliant with the new international consensus that favored free markets. The bank also worried that the housing policy might lead to social unrest owing to an increase in a segment of the urban population who lived under the constant threat of eviction in the cramped, insalubrious housing of the "spontaneous" housing sector, thus posing a threat to capitalist investment in the country.[22] Destruction of illegal housing eased in 1980, partly because of pressure from the World Bank, which feared the social consequences of the bulldozing, and the public housing corporations were privatized.

Urban policy widened the social divide between those who lived in legally secure, private or public housing and the rest who lived in legally precarious, informal housing, be it shantytowns or rogue "modern" subdivisions. Systematic destruction of informal housing in the 1970s, and more recently in the 1990s, has shown how these social divisions, shaped by state policy but exacerbated by economic hardship, amounted to a form of triage. Those who did not qualify to live in the city, either because they were too poor or did not have the political connections to stave off the bulldozers, were effectively razed out of urban existence.[23] Tactical forms of citizenship emerged in response to the eroded sovereignty of Côte-d'Ivoire in the face of powerful international organizations such as the World Bank.

Therapeutic Sovereignty

These historical examples of how people were typed highlight how criteria for classifying people may in fact exacerbate differences. Applying such criteria may even produce cleavages that did not previously exist in meaningful ways. Efforts to control HIV in Africa also rely on practices of naming (diagnosing), mapping (epidemiology), and grouping (HIV groups) something that did not "exist" as a tangible reality before. These efforts also seek to manage and affect the encounter between those who are HIV positive and those who are not. Conjugating a biopolitics of population with an anatomo-politics of the body, they are exemplars of biopower. Moreover, we have seen that efforts to address the epidemic introduced new forms of social differentiation and novel social cleavages that, in turn, led activists and people living with HIV to enact a therapeutic citizenship.

Long before the time of AIDS, the consolidation and exercise of colonial sovereignty made Côte-d'Ivoire a theater for practices of segregation and differentiation. Public health and housing policies sorted people into those who could live in the city and those who could not, separating Europeans from Africans in the early decades of the twentieth century, and rich from poor in the final decades. Bioracial distinctions gave way to ethnographic and eventually legal criteria. Colonial government made available systems of ethnic classification that generated economic and political cleavages along ethnic lines. A logic of sorting people according to administrative assumptions of value constituted a political calculus that balanced conflicting imperatives in the name of *sovereignty*. The colonial state sought to protect settlers and maximize the wealth it extracted from the colony, while the postcolonial state strove to modernize both economy and society while complying with the global rules that constrained its access to capital. In both cases these ambitions had to be weighed against the potential for political unrest, should these practices exclude too many people or those who were too valuable to alienate.

Practices for classifying people are often based on knowledge that is later revealed to be inaccurate or erroneous. Early segregation policies were based on the theory that diseases were caused by noxious vapors. Ethnographic knowledge glossed over some differences between groups while exaggerating others. Housing policy relied on inaccurate assumptions about local ways of life that were difficult to dispel, even when detailed surveys were carried out. Yet these practices, when implemented, turned knowledge into reality. Crowded into filthy shantytowns, Africans were sicker than Europeans. The use of ethnographic categories by the colonial state sharpened differences between groups and hardened ethnicity. Housing policy heightened economic differences, helped to produce an urban underclass, and fashioned citizenship. Fevers, "tribes," and bulldozers continue to haunt urban life.

As a lens for viewing the efforts to combat HIV in Burkina Faso and Côte-d'Ivoire, these historical examples tell us more. They suggest that the dividing practices and social categorizations used in efforts to control HIV might reveal themselves to have been crude in their reading of the social reality they sought to grasp—or might even be based on erroneous assumptions. These efforts may call into being social categories—in effect, kinds of people—that did not previously exist, in essence, "making up people."[24] Practices of differentiation may also result in unexpected consequences, enabling new forms of citizenship that become independent of the political calculus that gave birth to them. To recall the question that opened this chapter, what might be the consequences of this selective and partial exercise of biopower?

We have seen how therapeutic citizenship was fashioned from the ground up, in everyday life, as people confronted with HIV struggled to survive in the time of AIDS. Like the urban citizenship just discussed, these tactical forms of citizenship emerged through the exercise of biopower. Biopower constituted colonial sovereignty. With independence, national sovereignty channeled attempts to influence fate, enroll others in one's destiny, and shape the future. However, worsening political and economic conditions allowed international organizations like the World Bank to direct a biopolitics of the population. National sovereignty eroded. Might these attempts to manage populations and bodies with the imperative of controlling a deadly epidemic, the forms of citizenship that ensue, and the enactment of triage also erode national sovereignty? In its stead has not a *therapeutic sovereignty* emerged?

In the following chapter, I will further explore the political and economic crisis that struck Côte-d'Ivoire in the 1970s. It is here that a clearer picture emerges of how shifts in sovereignty produced new landscapes of constraint and increasingly located citizenship in the realm of self-fashioning.

THE CRISIS

....

Economies, Warriors, and the Erosion of Sovereignty

On 30 September 1969, large demonstrations held by "unemployed young men" led to mass arrests, the first warning sign that, even in good times, the "economic miracle" had generated a tide of rising expectations that were difficult to meet. Authorities dismissed the movement as an ethnic and xenophobic protest. The demonstrations were severely repressed, although eventually a quiet series of protracted negotiations and piecemeal reforms were undertaken (M. Cohen 1972). Coming at a time of high foreign investment and high economic growth, these first signs of the potential for political unrest deeply worried the government because of their potential effect on the economy. These concerns echoed those raised by the railway workers' strike of 1939, discussed in the previous chapter, and foreshadowed those expressed later by the World Bank. Political stability—or, more accurately, the perception of political stability—was seen as critical to the success of the foreign-investment-dominated economic model.[1] The decision by the authorities to cast what was an economic protest as an *ethnic* one showed the legacy of colonial ethnic cleavages in the political vocabulary of Côte-d'Ivoire and anticipated how future struggles would play out.

Although no one realized it at the time, the protests foreshadowed the gradual eclipse of Côte-d'Ivoire's sovereignty. This chapter examines the broader historical and social conditions that linked Côte-d'Ivoire's eroding sovereignty with increasing poverty and inequality.

It describes the rise and fall of a modern economy, the ensuing emergence of an "informal" economy, and the tactics that arose in the context of an unending economic crisis. Under these circumstances, where scarcity and diminishing prospects became the norm, a logic of rationing and competition emerged. In the language of the street, this was a time of "business" and "warriors," as youth grew up with the bitter realization that they would not enjoy the promise of a better future and aware that their lives had somehow been devalued in the face of economic crisis. I explore how citizenship mutated as, in the face of a disintegrating future, youth in Abidjan from the mid-1980s developed an urban culture that stressed self-fashioning in order to ensure survival. In the time of AIDS, triage is but a recent facet of a global dynamic of exclusion and expropriation that concentrates the violence of rationing on the most vulnerable.

James Ferguson's classic ethnography of the Zambian copperbelt (Ferguson 1999) describes the pervasive sense of disappointment and even bitterness that Zambians lived through—and continue to experience—as their economy disintegrated in the wake of the collapse of global copper prices. Like Zambia and other export-oriented economies, Côte-d'Ivoire suffered a similar fate. In Abidjan, however, rather than breeding a culture of disappointment, these unmet expectations led to an entrepreneurial urban culture. The self also became the subject of entrepreneurial remaking. I begin this chapter by describing this political economy, showing how political choices made far from Abidjan nonetheless shaped everyday life in the city. I then explore how those engagements, confronted with the inefficacy of political protest, ultimately took shape as tactics for disciplining body and mind in order to better confront a precarious economic reality. These tactics in effect constituted the self as an object of transformation. As technologies of the self, they provide a window onto the cultural logic of self-transformation that was already in place when AIDS and the efforts to combat it arrived. This cultural logic would go on to influence how people used the technologies of the self introduced by organizers of communities with HIV.

The Economic Crisis

The years after Côte-d'Ivoire's independence in 1961 coupled economic growth with massive state investments in public works, education, and housing. These investments expressed the promise that national sovereignty would herald entry into a modern society and finally make Ivoirians masters of their own destiny. This modernization was accompanied by broad social changes that many urban dwellers across the continent embraced, seeing in them the promise of a future of relative affluence and of greater possibilities for their children. Under the assault of the economic crisis of the 1980s, however, modernization crumbled and the state was no longer able to deliver on the "promissory notes" its program implied.[2] The gap widened between the expectations that Ivoirians developed in the context of modernity and the daunting challenges of everyday life.

The Ivoirian crisis first became evident in late 1978, with the collapse of coffee and cocoa prices on the global market.[3] Coffee and cocoa were introduced under colonial rule and formed the basis of the colony's plantation economy. Intensification of coffee and cocoa cultures was the central element of the postcolonial state's strategy for acquiring the foreign reserves it needed to pay for the international inputs essential to its modernization program. The impact of the drop in export prices spiraled into a full-blown crisis that year, as a second oil shock sent oil prices skyrocketing and increased the value of the U.S. dollar. Interest rates went through the roof, increasing the cost of servicing the Ivoirian debt. Côte-d'Ivoire was heavily dependent on exports to keep its modern economy functional. As a result, rising interest rates significantly deteriorated the balance of trade as more money flowed out for debt servicing than flowed in for exports. The Ivoirian government's sluggish response to the crisis, which, at the time, decision-makers thought was merely a temporary circumstance, only exacerbated the consequences of its worsening trade situation. When drought affected coffee and cocoa crops, falling agricultural outputs together with falling export prices and rising import prices brought down the heavily indebted economy like a house of cards.

Though the causes of the crisis were subject to intense debate, most observers agreed on the complexity of the interplay of situational and structural factors. Situational analyses focus on circumstances external to the Ivoirian economy (world commodity prices, interest rates, and so on) that led to the crisis. This was the view of the Ivoirian government, which saw itself as the victim of a chain of unfortunate circumstances. Structuralist economists, on the other hand, drew attention to structural weaknesses in the Ivoirian model: "Fundamental contradictions in the prevalent mode of accumulation, with enormous transfers from the agricultural sector to the foreign-dominated industrial sector" made it inevitable that external shocks would swamp the system (Fauré 1989, 71). Indeed, Marxist political economists used the

"Ivoirian model" as a case study in dependency theory. These studies argued that a small indigenous postcolonial planter class and an expatriate metropolitan (in this case largely French) bourgeoisie benefited from an "extractive," export-oriented economy. As a result, capital investment in the colony was kept to the minimum needed to extract resources with profits returning to the colonial center. The lack of further investment in the development of a local industrial base constituted a model of structurally "blocked" development (S. Amin 1967).

Structural Adjustment: An Economy Unravels

The structuralist analysis eventually proved largely correct (Campbell 1997). Indeed, the structural problem affected the entire global economic system, which favored the dependency of third-world economies and belied the promises that sovereignty had held for many newly decolonized nations. In Côte-d'Ivoire, the real crisis was in fact the collapse of the economic basis of the Ivoirian "miracle" in the new neoliberal global order that began to take hold from the 1970s. The realization that the problem ran deep was slow in coming. A fleeting economic upswing occurred in 1985, as favorable climatic conditions resulted in bumper coffee and cocoa crops. The cyclical nature of the cocoa crop and the vicissitudes of international capital markets, as well as the palliative effect of structural adjustment loans, masked the structural elements of the crisis. The dawning realization that the crisis might be permanent crept up throughout the 1980s. The Ivoirian government contracted with the World Bank at three-year intervals, starting in 1980, to implement structural adjustment policies as a condition of obtaining loans. These loans required a broad range of reforms that transformed the Ivoirian state's modernization program. These "conditionalities" played a major role in shaping the effect of the recession on Ivoirian society.

Côte-d'Ivoire was a "model pupil" (Duruflé 1988, 118) in implementing the conditions, exceeding the World Bank's targets. The loan in 1980 mandated a reduction in public investments from 25 percent to 16.5 percent of GDP over a three-year period. In 1983 the bank noted approvingly that the volume of public investment was down to 12 percent of GDP. This decrease translated into a massive 40 percent cut in public investments in real terms. By 1985, two years later, these cuts had increased to 70 percent (Duruflé 1988, 121). A second loan contracted in 1983 was more adventurous in its prescriptions. It ordered the diversification of the plantation economy into palm oil, rubber, and coconut and cautiously promoted the development of sugar, soybean, and irrigated rice production. These measures met with only partial economic success. The loan also stipulated reforms in state housing policy—most notably, rent increases through 1985—to reflect market values as well as major reductions in housing benefits for civil servants (Kanbur 1990, 11–14). Meanwhile, the government continued to obtain expensive credit in global equity markets based on overly optimistic predictions, recycling its debt and in effect "borrowing from Peter to pay Paul." This increased the drain on the state's finances when expected economic growth did not materialize (Duruflé 1988, 120–24). Côte-d'Ivoire defaulted on its loan payments for the first time in 1987.

Despite being a model pupil, structural adjustment did not deliver the promised dividends. Commenting on "the disproportion between the results obtained in terms of debt relief, and the costs, measured in terms of deflation, divestment, and decreases in social services," Gilles Duruflé, an economist with the French Ministry of Cooperation, attributed the failure of structural adjustment to the limits of the mode of political and economic accumulation that had characterized the Ivoirian miracle (Duruflé 1988, 141). By the early 2000s, a consensus had emerged that it was the structural adjustment policies themselves that had failed to achieve their economic goals and had in fact worsened social conditions in countries that were forced to apply them.[4] The World Bank has, since 2002, emphasized that poverty reduction strategies be included as a goal of governments' receiving loans, an implicit acknowledgment of the role of earlier structural adjustment in worsening poverty.[5]

The Contradictory Effects of Structural Adjustment

While certain effects of the conditionalities were felt immediately, others took longer to register in the social fabric. Decreased public inputs shrank the formal economy by 30 percent as the state reduced salaries and froze hiring. The effect of this cannot be overexaggerated. The state was by far the country's largest formal employer and paid high salaries. The preponderance of French bureaucrats and technical advisers who stayed on after independence artificially inflated salaries. Earning good incomes in the formal sector, civil servants redistributed income through extended kinship networks, both in the city and the country.[6] As a result of structural adjustment, urban per capita income decreased by 45 percent between 1978 and 1985 (Duruflé 1988; see table 1 below). The economy entered a deflationary spiral, short-circuiting a strategy that hoped to increase government revenue by stimulating economic

TABLE 1   Progression of poverty in Côte-d'Ivoire, as measured by economic indices, 1959–95

Index	1959	1970	1979	1985	1988	1993	1995
GNP per capita			396	314	281	234	226
Private consumption per capita			225	189	187	148	129
Incidence of poverty				11.1	17.8	32.3	36.8
Intensity of poverty				2.9	4.5	9.0	10.4
Severity of poverty				1.3	1.7	3.4	3.2
Gini coefficient	0.46	0.53	0.61	0.39	0.35	0.37	0.35
Income share of lowest quintile as %	6.6	3.9	2.1	5.4	7.3	7.1	7.5

Adapted from World Bank 1996, 9. Figures are expressed in thousands of CFAs, at constant 1987 prices. The intensity of poverty index "measures the percentage shortfall in aggregate consumption of the poor below the poverty line. Thus in 1995, the intensity of poverty index was 0.84, implying that to raise the consumption level of each poor individual exactly up to the poverty line of CFA 144,800 would require a sum equivalent to 10.4% of the poverty line multiplied by the total population. In theory, a perfectly targeted subsidy to the poor of this amount could enable all minimum consumption needs to be met. This is equivalent to 5–6% of GDP, a very substantial gap. . . . The severity index is a weighted index of poverty giving the greatest weight to those who are poorest" (World Bank 1996, 9–10). The gini coefficient measures the degree of economic inequality in a society by measuring the gap between actual distribution of incomes and an ideal income distribution; the higher the number, the more inequality, and vice versa. A perfectly egalitarian society would have a Gini coefficient of 0.

growth through the liberalization of the economic sector. The crisis, as shown by the figures below, was nothing short of an economic tsunami. It left in its wake poverty of unprecedented scale and intensity.

A somewhat conflicting picture emerges from the data concerning the overall effect of structural readjustment and the economic crisis. Macroeconomic indicators suggest that income disparities grew during the boom years, only to be compressed with the crisis. However, "all three indices of poverty — incidence, intensity and severity . . . increased consistently over the 1985–1995 period of the crisis. Collectively, the indices point to a rapidly building crisis" (World Bank 1996, 8–9, table 5.1). In other words, the boom years benefited the wealthy more than the poor. With the recession, the wealthy lost proportionately more income. For those less well off, relatively smaller losses plunged many into a spiral of poverty. Another paradox is that although macroeconomic indicators of social inequality (the Gini coefficients and the poorest quintile's share of national GDP, noted in table 1) improved during the crisis, social scientists working in Abidjan reported worsening inequality.[7] How to explain this contradiction? The answer lies in how structural adjustment refracted inequalities in housing and schooling.

Housing

The legacy of colonial and postcolonial housing policy played an important role in mediating the impact of the economic crisis and the structural adjustment it entailed. This was because housing was used as capital for negotiating an increasingly uncertain economic environment. At the behest of the World Bank, Côte-d'Ivoire privatized government housing in order to allow market forces to operate freely in the previously subsidized modern housing market. As a result, citizens' access to housing capital tightened. With these reforms, a significant margin of the "middle classes" who had aspired to modern housing were no longer able to afford market rates and were forced into the informal housing sector. Initially, municipal services to what were previously considered shantytowns improved with the influx of new, less marginalized residents who were better connected to those in power. This observation, along with the fact that the state ceased to bulldoze illegal neighborhoods in 1989, was taken as an indication of the new political clout of the residents of these informal neighborhoods.[8] It is more likely, however, that it reflected the fact that even the well connected were pressured by the economic crisis into the precarious housing sector (Le Pape, Vidal, and Yapi-Diahou 1991). This situation constituted a tacit recognition that the goals of the urban plans of the 1960s and 1970s — modern housing for a largely middle-class urban population — had been abandoned.

The shift in housing policy appears to have actually deepened social inequality *within* the middle class, though this was not its intent. Those who had purchased subsidized housing were largely able to preserve their economic status, compensating for revenue shortfalls by renting out property. Those who did not own property were economically vulnerable to rising rents as state subsidies were removed. As job and salary cuts came about, these individuals found themselves impoverished (Vidal 1997). In other words, the already fragile middle class splintered: those with property were well positioned to take advantage of subsequent economic growth because of the capital they were able to preserve, while those who were not property owners were no longer shielded from market rental rates by state housing subsidies. As a result, these people found themselves more exposed to poverty.

The economic crisis revealed paradoxical effects of the state's housing policy, which was intended as a lever to improve access to a middle-class life even for those less well-off. Instead, it constituted a subsidy to the wealthier that paid off in times of recession. The end to subsidies, mandated by structural adjustment, was meant to level the playing field for the poor, but in times of economic recession, liberalizing the housing market increased the ranks of the poor, as they were less able to shield themselves from the rising cost of living.

Deschooling

With structural adjustment, investments in educational establishments were drastically curtailed, as state funding for the educational sector was scaled back.[9] Enrollments declined because the combination of school fees and the loss of faith in the value of diplomas meant that parents were more selective in choosing which children to send to school. Girls were disproportionately affected. This effectively "deschooled" a generation of youth, who went to primary school but had little access to schooling beyond the sixth grade. This change was reflected in the decline of gross educational rates (the proportion of the population of school age that had ever been to school: see table 2).

While most children attended primary school, bottlenecks in sixth and tenth grades mean that many children were not able to continue beyond these stages. Statistics collected by the Ministry of Education indicated that the number of students passing into sixth grade decreased gradually from 45 percent at independence, to stabilize at roughly 15 percent at the end of the 1970s. The decline in passages into sixth grade was a reflection of a huge increase in intake of students in the period just after independence. The cohort of children entering the system began to shrink in the mid-1960s, a trend that continued with the crisis. As a result, the proportion entering sixth grade stabilized until the crisis hit. Entry into tenth grade was directly affected by the crisis: admissions fell precipitously from over 50 percent just before the crisis to roughly 10 percent by 1994 (Proteau 1997). The social consequences were enormous. Partially schooled youth nonetheless believed in the promise of a better future, a hope that lingered long after the crisis, nourished by memories

TABLE 2 Gross educational rates in percentages

1985–86	1988–89	1989–90	1990–91	1991–92	1992–93
74.5	72.8	71.8	69.1	67.7	66

Source: Adapted from Proteau 1997, 639.

of the flush times of the economic miracle. As a result, new generations grew up feeling cheated of the promise of modernity, particularly because they believed that education was the path to a better life.

Three reasons account for the apparent contradiction between social science accounts of *increasing* inequality and economic data that measured *decreasing* social inequality in the period of structural adjustment that followed the crisis. First, *perceptions* of inequality changed. As the crisis dashed expectations, those who were worse off, realizing that the chances their situation might improve were nonexistent, became more sensitive to inequality. Second, responses to the crisis were heterogeneous. The crisis separated the wheat from the chaff, as some managed to improvise tactics for preserving income while others did not. Anecdotal and ethnographic data confirmed World Bank economists' findings that a "lucky few," even among the poor, were able to preserve their assets (Grootaert and Kanbur 1995). As a result, different outcomes occurred *within* social groups, as neighbors and friends were only too aware. Third, in addition to these experiential reasons for the heightened sensitivity to social inequality during the crisis, the fault lines traced by housing policy fractured with the economic stress of the crisis. Frustration grew within the "subaltern" social class that had previously defined itself relative to a monolithic and ostentatious nationalist élite. The "little people" became "paupers" (Vidal 1990). The mechanisms that refracted inequality within social groups allowed the "lucky few" to weather the economic crisis more successfully and were instrumental in further fracturing the population along economic lines. An urban culture of "getting by" resulted.

No School, What Future?

What happened to the generations of deschooled youth who stayed in the city? As the economic crisis deepened into a recession, many families expected children to pull their weight by contributing financially to family meals. Those that did not were expected to eat elsewhere. By the mid-1970s, as many as a third of the children in Côte-d'Ivoire were *confiés*, or placed with relatives in the city (Étienne 1979). This was usually because urban relatives were considered wealthier and therefore more able to support the schooling of rural children. The schooling crisis partially reversed the flow of child placement from urban back to rural areas. Since children were too much of a burden—because they got into trouble on the street or were unable to support themselves—they were often sent up-country, either to live with relatives or to return to their parents in rural areas. Among those who stayed in the city, however, many joined the informal economy, some as apprentices or to learn manual trades, while others went into *affaires*, or "business." This usage corresponds to the popular term "hustling," which one informant succinctly explained to me was "what you've gotta go out and do every day to survive your life." The expression refers to engaging in the commerce of goods obtained by unorthodox means or in confidence schemes. Others took up the *petit metiers* (odd jobs) that the city is famous for (Touré 1985). As Marc Le Pape (1986, 112) notes, hustling implied a set of skills: the art of relations, social dexterity, or a capital of aptitudes and social resources. Access to primary school modernized youth by giving them literacy skills and generating expectations of a place in society. While some returned to the village, the majority of these youth swelled the ranks of those in the urban parallel economy.

The effects of change in the education system extended further than simply excluding some from pursuing their studies. Prior to the crisis, university studies were free, and students who passed the *baccalauréat* received bursaries and numerous other benefits. This reflected the Ivoirian state's desire to invest in creating an élite class. Those that were educated could take over the mantle of the state's institutions from the French bureaucrats who continued to hold the reins of state after independence.

As salary freezes and increasing workloads decreased the spending power of teachers, selection for entry into higher classes became less dependent on academic merit alone. *Le couloir* (connections), bribes, and even sexual favors emerged as tactics that could secure academic promotion.[10] This added to the financial burden imposed by school fees, a mechanism of cost recovery that structural adjustment imposed in Côte-d'Ivoire and indeed throughout the developing world. As a result, educational success became increasingly dependent on students' ability to translate social, financial, and occasionally even sexual capital into better grades. The latter was humorously referred to as "MST" (*moyennes sexuellement transmises*, or sexually transmitted grades) (Proteau 1997, 651), a parody based on the French acronym commonly used to refer to sexually transmitted diseases (*maladies sexuellement transmises*).[11] Youth developed a variety of tactics for raising money from and making connections with relatives. Flowery letters to senior brothers were perhaps most typical of this genre, part of a repertoire of skills developed to earn income (Le Pape 1986).

Since continuation in school required being able to borrow from relatives and connections, youth were increasingly dependent on kin. This process has been documented by a broad ethnographic study of youth in Abidjan, coordinated by French anthropologist Alain Marie (1997a), which reveals the difficulties of negotiating between urban life, with its culture of individualism driven by schooling and mass media, and village life, with its more collective forms of belonging. Youth, most of whom were born or at least grew up in the city, were apprehensive of village life and the consequences of increased dependence on the extended kinship network of the village for their schooling. They feared being clasped by a suffocating embrace, explaining to Marie's team of anthropologists the dangers of witchcraft from jealous or resentful family members. Witchcraft accusations and fears of witchcraft became idioms through which the oppressiveness of increased dependence on kinship relations was expressed, and it exercised a powerful force, countering the individualizing tendency of urban life (Marie 1997b).

With the advent of the crisis, the horizons of possibility, which had seemed so vast at the time of independence, became increasingly constrained. For youth who could no longer continue their schooling, or students who could no longer expect a job upon graduation, the disappointment was particularly cruel. For many of these young people, the inability to establish an economically stable situation condemned them to a kind of perpetual social adolescence. Unable to become economically self-sufficient—and hence to marry—they could not be recognized as true adults in either "traditional" or "modern" terms. Youth excluded from the formal economy grew increasingly disenchanted and embittered as the years of crisis dragged on. Nonetheless, despite the crisis, the city promised much, illuminated by the bright lights of its popular culture, media, and lure of wealth. In this context, perceptions of the economy as a zero-sum game, whereby one can win only at the expense of another, began to take hold, paralleling the rise of an "informal" economy even as the formal one unraveled.

Rise of a Parallel Economy

In the wake of the economic crisis that began in the late 1970s, what was at the time referred to as an "informal economy" in Abidjan "exploded" between 1980 and 1985 (Haeringer 1988). Abidjan began to look like other African cities. The sterile appearance of its throughways receded as sidewalks and roadways grew crowded with ambulatory vendors and impromptu businesses of every kind. It seemed as though the crisis had unleashed a previously unsuspected entrepreneurial zest and creative spirit. *Maquis*, informal bars previously cloistered in courtyards in the colonial tradition, spilled out onto sidewalks, and older corner boutiques diversified. For modernization theorists, the informal economy represents a transitional stage from subsistence-oriented, traditional economic forms to more "mature," capitalist modes of accumulation. As a result, informal economies were little studied until the 1970s. However, their growing economic dynamism belied the predictions of the modernization theorists and heralded a spate of studies throughout the developing world. More recently, an anthropological scholarship has preferred the term "parallel" economy to better reflect the fact that it is, in fact, highly organized.[12]

In Abidjan, studies have identified a bewildering array of trades, practices, and savoir faire. Indeed, it seems that no aspect of everyday life was left untouched by the informal economy, as a bewildering array of goods and services were traded. The trades that were exercised within the informal economy extended from barbers, tailors, carpenters, gardeners, hair braiders, and car washers, to car parkers, traffic managers, card plastifiers, water resellers, light-bulb repairers, foot washers, soothsayers, group psychotherapists, nail clippers, cell-phone reprogrammers, and ambulatory bankers. This was in addition to merchants selling all kind of goods imaginable. Two crucial observations emerged from these studies of the informal economy. The first was its striking innovation. The majority of the trades practiced were highly individualized, both in the way skills were deployed and in the imagination with which market niches were carved out. The second was that economic success was highly dependent on the ability to maintain and "read" social networks. In an economy where liquidity was in short supply, economic success involved knowing to whom it was possible to extend credit, for how much, and for how long. Merchants who extended too much credit were unable to recover debts and stood to lose money; those who extended too little credit could not generate sufficient turnover for their business to be viable. In addition to skillful manipulation of credit, merchants relied on social networks for other business fundamentals. Social networks furnished the market intelligence to determine the value of goods and set prices that were competitive and yet could still generate healthy profit margins. Networks also decreased transaction costs by allowing retailers to have a "direct line" to wholesalers, producers or importers; conversely, social networks translated into distribution networks for wholesalers.

Success in the informal economy therefore required a broad range of skills. These encompassed the invention and practice of innovative trades and the maintenance of social relations. Success required that discipline, procedures, and analysis be applied to one's self. From the mid-1970s on, youth sought to secure a future in an uncertain economic climate through self-fashioning, as I will explore in further detail below.[13]

The Urban Culture of Self-Fashioning

Population growth, which swelled the ranks of the young, exacerbated the potential for political unrest when the crisis began in 1979. By then, it had been made clear that in Côte-d'Ivoire's one-party state, open political dissidence was frowned upon. The disenchantment that resulted was channeled into underground political activities that would eventually culminate in multiparty politics in 1989. Urban cultural forms, such as *zouglou* dance and music,[14] expressed this disaffection but were later appropriated by the state as emblematic of Ivoirian national culture.

A strong undercurrent of protest found expression in myriad cultural forms—mainly popular music and dance—that signaled the emergence of an urban culture centered on the social reality of Abidjan. This popular culture was wedded to the growth of the informal economy that characterized the popular response to the economic crisis. The lingua franca of this urban culture is Nouchi, an Abidjanais dialect. Nouchi combines French, English, and mainly Dioula words within a syntax poor in prepositions and articles, which its speakers describe as "African." Recalling the multiethnic nature of Abidjan and the extraordinary proportion of migrants, French was, and still is, the dominant common language. Dioula, a language of traders spoken in markets, comes a distant second. My informants recalled that Nouchi, although no one called it that at the time, was already widely spoken in the 1970s. Their awareness of its distinctiveness came from school, where it was

Lang outside state

forbidden and they were at times punished when they spoke it. Nouchi became the linguistic vehicle for the youth culture of Abidjan.

The expansion of *le parler d'Abidjan* (the language of Abidjan) was linked to both the crisis and the development of the informal economy in multiple ways. Partial schooling and high literacy rates originally reinforced French as the lingua franca in this multiethnic city, as no African language achieved national status in the manner of Mooré in Burkina Faso, Swahili in Tanzania, or Wolof in Sénégal. This was for both demographic and political reasons, as no ethnic group was dominant in the city, and French was the language of modernization. In addition, the demographic preponderance of youth—as in many developing countries, over half the population is below eighteen years of age—helped to disseminate the linguistic innovations of youth culture. The ethnic and linguistic heterogeneity of the city extended into its neighborhoods. Although in parts of the city certain groups predominated, the mobility of urban dwellers across the different sections of the city precluded the development of linguistic enclaves. Because it was in these mobile elements that Nouchi and, by extension, the cultural vernacular of urban life emerged, this is where it is possible to best understand how, in the absence of formal education, self-fashioning was a powerful tool for confronting economic uncertainty and keeping alive ideals of progress and the good life.

Collecting Fares

Gbaka, a Nouchi word whose origins are unknown, refers to Abidjan's private twenty-seat minibuses.[15] Gbakas have existed in the city since the late colonial period. In 1960, the city's urban transit corporation Société des Transports Abidjanais (SOTRA) was formed to respond to the transportation needs of a growing population in a growing urban area. Initially, although SOTRA had a small rolling stock of Renault buses and, technically, a monopoly on public transportation, the private gbakas were tolerated. By 1974, however, SOTRA was well equipped with secondhand buses from French cities. Gbakas, deemed a nuisance because of the recklessness of their drivers, were banned from the city core. With structural adjustment, however, SOTRA had difficulty recovering its costs and keeping its aging fleet on the road. Breakdowns were legion, and delays became commonplace. The company was unable to respond to the transportation needs generated by the explosive growth of the townships of Abobo and Yopougon (now estimated to have between one and two million inhabitants each), both of which are over ten kilometers from the central Plateau district. As a result, a fleet of gbakas once again moved in to fill the gap in serving these sprawling townships, encouraged by the World Bank's emphasis on liberalization of the transportation sector in the late 1980s.

The profession of gbaka fare-collector—the term used is *apprenti*—is one that has largely been taken up by deschooled youth. It is an example of how self-fashioning may translate into economic power. These youths were often in their late teens and early twenties on average and were a fixture of every-day life in the city in the 1990s. Most noticeable as they dangle out of open doors, sucking their teeth loudly and rhythmically shouting out destinations, these youth are often credited with disseminating Nouchi throughout the city. The staccato of destination calls, punctuated by announcements of the num-ber of seats available, is Nouchi's metronome and rhyme, the beat of city life. Nouchi's cultural versatility is best appreciated as apprentis squeeze through a crowded gbaka, bills curled between their fingers, collecting fares and making small talk. This habitus and speed is emblematic of the urban culture of the city; but it is also the product of hard-earned skills that have been picked up on the street. In the face of adversity, these youths have turned urban culture into a viable skill that is *embodied*.

Interviews I conducted with apprentis in 1999 led me to estimate that the number of youth that engaged in this occupation was significant, perhaps in the tens of thousands. (Many worked part-time and moved in and out of this line of work, making estimates difficult.) Reputed to be "*petits loubards*" or rogues, many of these youth actually lived with their families and contrib-uted economically to the household. Apprentis actually earned a significant income, averaging six thousand CFA per day (roughly fifteen dollars), which was three times the average income for unskilled work. Apprentis get to keep whatever fares they collect after the gbaka has left its originating station— hence the economic motivation that explains their assiduity in beckoning, cajoling, seducing, and even pulling passengers onto moving vehicles. The work is difficult and dangerous—agility, coordination, and stamina must be accompanied by social skills. Apprentis must know how to "speak properly" with passengers and have a repertoire of techniques for scanning the crowds that pullulate along the roadside in order to detect potential passengers, get their attention, and entice them on board.

Some apprentis saved their incomes, investing it in bank accounts at local *Caisses populaires*, or credit unions.[16] With these savings, some of these youth dreamed of paying the fees necessary for getting a driver's license and, with a driver's income, eventually saving up enough to buy their own gbaka. These youths translated faith in credit unions, the stability of the state, and the value of money into pragmatic, everyday economic tactics. Some had succeeded: they were the "lucky few"—very few indeed—for whom apprenti-ship can translate into social stability. For most, however, individuality was expressed in the maquis of the rue Princesse, the blaring hotspot in Central Yopougon, where they could dance to zouglou until dawn and where they spent their money on beer and women. Gbakas are a social technology, generating a matrix of experience for both operators (the apprentis) and users—just like the telephone help lines discussed in chapter 2.

Bodybuilding

"Real" loubards—roughnecks—also form part of the social landscape of the city, and they are yet another example of the embodiment of self-fashioning. The stocky young men who led opposition to Houphouët in the late 1980s and early 1990s, and before that in the 1969 "sans travail" demonstrations, were said to be Bété. The Bété were a diverse group of "tribes" in the southwest of the country who were fused into one ethnic group by the French colonial administration. Their reputation as quarrelsome likely originated in colonial times, when French policy encouraged "allogène" (of foreign origin) Baoulé planters to develop plantations in Bété country. The Baoulé, migrants with a kinship structure that had been adapted to the plantation mode of production, consolidated their plantations and were more successful than the Bété. The smaller Bété plantations demonstrated a more rigid lineage-based mode of production (Hecht 1984). The Bété also had competition from the west, because the Kru from Liberia were encouraged to develop plantations on their land. These diffuse rivalries and struggles over land crystallized as a Bété rivalry to the Baoulé who, once Houphouët was made president, became the politically dominant ethnic group (Dozon 1985a). Labeling dissenters as Bété followed easily and reflected the ease with which political struggle could be parsed along ethnic lines by Ivoirian authorities who, wittingly or not, drew on a colonial logic of divide-and-rule.[17] These divisions would continue to haunt Côte-d'Ivoire's First Republic.

Despite the connotations of criminality and public disorder that attach to them, the private security industry employs many loubards. Certainly, the sight of intimidating, generously muscled young men patrolling in front of

Abidjan's chic shops and nightclubs is a common one. This niche of the parallel economy was not considered glamorous. It was not a "modern" office job, but nonetheless, it was better than being unemployed. A subculture of bodybuilding was tied into this professional category. Free weights, barbell racks, and bench presses, ingeniously engineered from recycled auto parts, were used by youths in impromptu gyms I visited. Special diets were consumed, with the hope that a well-developed physique would allow those that ingested them to appear sufficiently intimidating to get a job as a bouncer at a nightclub. The wage for a bouncer was average for unskilled labor: fifty thousand to sixty thousand CFA, or one hundred dollars, monthly. This was just enough to pay for rent, food, medicines, and the occasional night out. Being a bouncer also offered the opportunity for tips, especially from patrons who feel they might not otherwise gain entry.

Like others in the informal economy, these loubards were "deschooled"— but literate, and this had important implications. The crisis of the 1980s ushered in an era of "insecurity" in the 1990s, as armed crime became rampant. Abidjan developed a reputation for danger, rivaled only by Nigeria's large cities (Marguerat 1998). The stark realities of cheek-to-jowl inequality had always been there, but with growing crime the wealthy became increasingly nervous about the potential for danger. As a result, private security became a booming industry. Initially, most firms were French owned, but enterprising *vigils*—as security guards are known—set up and expanded their own firms. Many of these entrepreneurs drew on skills and contacts acquired during military or police service. The high literacy of the work force meant that these firms were able to professionalize easily.

Cultivating one's body to become a bodyguard could also yield a ticket to France. Through the 1990s, the growth of marginalized immigrant communities in the vast suburban developments ringing Paris was paralleled by a growth in petty—and occasionally violent—crime and youth gangs modeled on American inner-city "gangsta" culture. Consequently, the market for private security has been a rapidly growing one in metropolitan France, one that cannot easily be met with French labor alone. As a result, over 170 Ivoirian private security firms had branches in the greater Paris area by 2000. These security firms offered expertise in security, but also a ready supply of cheaply paid, largely illegal, African labor.[18] In addition to being cheap, literate, and muscled labor, Abidjanais security guards had the added advantage of knowing urban street culture, and were therefore assumed to be better able to "reason" with their "*black et beur*" (Black and Arab) French "brothers." The reality was, of course, not so simple. Parisian gangs did not look on eager security agents kindly, particularly when their zeal resulted in local gang members being hauled off to the local *Commissariat* (precinct). For the undocumented Ivoirian security guards, vengeance was a common, and occasionally deadly, consequence of this line of work. But for young Ivoirian men still in Abidjan, the chance to go to France promised the dream of a better future. Leaving Abidjan for Paris was not a simple affair, however. Visas and papers could always be arranged but required the right contacts who could assist with visa form preparations, supply the required documents, and coach potential immigrants in how to pass interviews with French officials. For those with a modicum of schooling and the ability to fashion their bodies into an intimidating physique, immigration offered the best chance of material success.

Hustling

For those whose bodies or minds did not direct them into guarding or manual labor, les affaires—"hustling"—was another option. Some who got into this line of work had obtained their baccalaureat, or had even been able to attend university. Others had been "deschooled" because they never obtained the grades to finish high school. Considered "intellectuals" by other youths because of their schooling, they were not considered apt for manual work, or for hawking goods on the side of the road.

In a city where stark inequalities are painfully juxtaposed, a seemingly endless array of get-rich-quick scams appealed to "good-lookin," "fast-talkin" youth. These all required "hustlers" to earn a wealthy person's trust, usually by offering that person a chance to earn money easily with a minimum investment, while at the same time appearing naïve and unaware of the actual potential of the scheme. The wealthy person is duped into making the initial investment and then strung along until the trickster vanishes with the money. As one informant told me, the scam works "because they are greedy, and they think other black people are stupid while they are smart because they are rich." Methods for gaining the investor's confidence included using bank accounts, dummy corporations, "black money" (suitcases of U.S. dollars soaked in black ink that can be removed with a special solvent), and a slew of business plans.

For others, religion offered the possibility of salvation in the here-and-now. Preaching was a potentially lucrative profession, as the profusion of

Abidjan's impromptu churches shows. As one informant explained to me, "It depends on which environment you've been in. Those that go to church and are smart figure out how it works . . . you know, most of their preaching is based on give, give, give . . . and here you have a bunch of poor people turning to God to improve their situation and all you've got to do is, say, give two cents here or three cents there and you've got a thousand of them in your church and you figure it out, you've got four thousand dollars at the end of the day." The potential for small contributions to multiply into considerable sums became most visible with the advent of the Brazilian Pentecostal "Universal Church of the Kingdoms of God" in Abidjan. This church bought up all the local neighborhood cinemas and converted them into halls of worship in the late 1990s. The cinemas were packed day and night as back-to-back sermons succeeded each other, accompanied by exhortations for contributions. This would inevitably reach a frenzy, with worshippers throwing in fistfuls of bills—sums that had to be carted out, it was rumored, in trucks.

What exactly characterized youths who "made it" in these urban, African capitalist practices? Intelligence, being articulate, and being "good-looking" were prerequisites. Being "good-looking" did not refer to physical attributes but rather to looking the part, looking trustworthy, upright, honest. In addition to being "good-looking," one also had to be "open to other cultures" and have experienced many different *milieux* or subcultures. This was something, I was told, that comes "with traveling." The ability to master technologies of persuasion, as a hustler or a preacher, was explained as largely a product of circumstances, of a path settled into after the trials-and-errors of trying to survive in a succession of African cities.

Conclusion: Tactics and Social Relations

The economic crisis of the 1980s and the structural adjustment policies imposed by the World Bank were powerful drivers of social differentiation, deepening poverty and economic division. These political and economic conditions eroded national sovereignty. The effects were refracted through the prism of urban protest, youth culture, and the parallel economy. Survival, particularly for deschooled youth, required becoming a "street warrior," versed in the art of reading social relations (knowing whom to trust), the arts of persuasion (whose confidence might be earned and how), or the ability to transform one's self (through religion, or through bodybuilding).[19] Navigating the complex and increasingly differentiated social reality of the city required the body to be disciplined and the mind sharpened. The tools to do this constituted technologies of the self. Alongside practices that fashioned identity through ethnic categories and kinship relations, technologies of the self fostered self-transformation in order to meet the challenges of a rapidly changing society in the throes of economic turmoil. At times, people used these technologies of the self with explicit goals in mind, for example, getting to France or purchasing a vehicle. At other times, self-fashioning was engaged less purposefully, as a way to pass time, assuage the suffering of poverty, or indulge in the pleasures of selfhood. As part of the pragmatics of urban life, these technologies both expressed and constituted the self as an object of transformation. Technologies of the self palliated the inability of citizenship to offer the promise of a better future in an era of structural adjustment and eroding national sovereignty.

Scholars have already argued that structural adjustment—and the political and economic precariousness it created in many parts of the developing world—contributed to making people vulnerable to HIV. Poverty and social inequality, they have shown, forced women to trade sex for money. Crumbling health systems were not able to control other sexually transmitted diseases that fuelled the spread of HIV.[20] Instead of rehearsing these well-established arguments, this chapter has explored other ways in which political and economic conditions shaped the epidemic. Mass impoverishment and the sharpening of social inequality generated new social practices for surviving in times of scarcity, shrinking prospects, and diminishing national sovereignty. Despite their diversity, these strategies shared a common feature: survival required self-transformation. The self-help groups, testimonials, and counseling practices that proliferated in the wake of the AIDS epidemic joined the armamentarium required for survival. The pragmatics of survival in a "zero-sum" social and economic battleground was one of competition (see for instance Kirschke 2000). On this battleground, intimate disclosures—such as those that the AIDS campaigns elicited—could be used as weapons. This will be the subject of the next chapter.

USES AND PLEASURES
....

The Republic Inside Out

The effort to combat HIV produced a market for testimonials of HIV-positive people. Confessional technologies were used to train people to "come out" and disclose secrets about sex and illness. This chapter explores the linkages between sex, intimate disclosures, and social relations in the years leading up to and during the time of AIDS in Côte-d'Ivoire. As we have seen in the stories of Abdoulaye, Issa, Jeanne, and others, in the 1990s AIDS testimonials were promoted to empower people living with HIV and foster solidarity. These disclosures were elicited in order to solidify social bonds and for use as a weapon in the battle against HIV. However, we also saw that this technology of the self had unintended consequences and, in some cases, ended up disrupting social ties and creating divisions where none had previously existed. The disclosures incited to "give a face" to the epidemic were public confessions. They served as moral barometers, and whether they nurtured solidarity or fostered jealousy depended on the moral anxieties of the time. Confessions were a double-edged sword. As economic contraction and social fragmentation fostered a zero-sum logic of competition in Côte-d'Ivoire, disclosures about sex and sexuality could be used as technologies of persuasion, or even as weapons against powerful people. This wielding of words further emphasizes the ambivalence of disclosure in the time of AIDS. Indeed, the fault lines traced by earlier forms of triage and the value placed on personal secrets and their revelation in a deteriorating political and economic climate set the stage for an explosion of political violence.

The "War of the Sexes"

The way people talk about sex in Abidjan reflects the city's demographic and economic history. This history is crucial to understanding the shape disclosures about sex would have in the time of AIDS, from the 1990s on. Until the 1950s, the population of Abidjan (like other African cities) was still largely made up of young male migrants from the countryside.[1] At the time, fetchingly dressed young women were scorned and viewed as prostitutes by many.[2] Rounded up by the police, they were often forced to undergo speculum exams and administered vaginal disinfectants (Vidal 1979). In her landmark studies of sexuality in Abidjan, Claudine Vidal (1977, 1980) chronicles how the city in the 1970s gradually "sweetened," as elegant women, clad in Western and African fashions, sporting new hairstyles, and exhibiting seductive behavior, became part of everyday life. This did not pass unnoticed, either by the men it "inflamed," or in hit songs, gossip, and advice columns of Abidjan's dailies that chronicled everyday life in the city during this period. The newspapers—and the public that read them—were preoccupied with the new sexual liberalization, the brazenness of *lycéénnes* (high-school girls), and the potent mix of seduction, money, and power. "Where else could ministers be seen in their Mercedes outside schoolyards?" they asked (as cited in Vidal 1977).

Vidal (1979) also chronicled the interest that the appearance of such "ultra-modern" women sparked in the popular culture of the city. Was the widespread Abidjanais practice of keeping a mistress or two the modernization of polygamy, and hence acceptable in the name of African values? Or was it a threat to the African family? Why were such women so desirable to men? Because mistresses were assumed to divide their time between several lovers, they were thought to be "liberated" rather than exploited. Economic barriers to having mistresses were resented. If one was a "big man," with a car and a government job, there were no obstacles, but for the "little men," laborers and lowly clerks, things were not so easy. At the time, the discourse on mistresses was remarkably gendered, expressing male anxieties about the rapid pace of social change wrought by postcolonial economic growth and urbanization. There was little discussion of how wives viewed these developments. Husbands professed the traditional ideas of family responsibility, which conveniently only required handing over enough money to keep food on the table and pay school expenses for children. The rest, wives bitterly complained, went to the upkeep of mistresses. Conscious of their tenuous hold over their husbands, wives developed their own strategies for achieving economic independence. During the colonial period, women had engaged in a lively commerce as purveyors of palm wine and keepers of informal watering holes hidden away from colonial authorities in private courtyards. In the years of the economic miracle, women continued to pioneer businesses in a small and largely invisible parallel economy (Vidal 1977, 1991). In the 1970s, they started businesses out of the family home to supplement the income their husbands earned in the modern, formal sector of the economy.

When the economic crisis hit, as husbands lost their "real" jobs in the formal economy, the balance of power in the household shifted, and male anxieties took an ominous turn. Women were economically empowered, relative to their husbands, as shown by data that female-headed households weathered the recession better than male-headed households. In addition to growing female participation in the parallel economy, serial surveys indicated that the proportion of women who were active in the workforce increased from 29 percent to 49 percent between 1979—the year the economic crisis hit—and 1992 (Kanbur 1990). Women demanded a greater say in things. The debate was acrimonious, an escalation of gendered tensions that had already begun in the years of the Ivoirian economic miracle in the 1960s and 1970s. Vidal reports that wives began to demand accountability from husbands, and men sometimes responded with violence, in what she called a "war of the sexes" (Vidal 1977).

Since Abidjan was a self-consciously ultramodern and Westernized city, it is not surprising that a discourse of sexuality, marked by concern over "sexual liberalization," emerged there more forcefully than elsewhere in the region (Le Pape and Vidal 1984). In the 1970s and early 1980s changing gender roles were widely discussed. In the moral imagination, sexuality served as a barometer of social and economic changes. Talk about sex was linked to economic changes and freighted with anxieties about the new inequalities these introduced.

Sex, Power, and Money

In Abidjan's popular culture of the 1970s, discussions of homosexuality focused on "aesthetics," pleasure, and milieu. For instance, a popular drag show at the time drew attention in newspaper stories that, while alluding to homosexuality, focused on the aesthetics of the show and highlighted the city's sexual modernism (Nguyen 2005). In the wake of the economic crisis, talk about sex was once again a moral barometer. Homosexuality became the subject of informal conversations and rumors that linked sex between men to issues of power and money. By the mid-1990s, graphic representations of homosexual sex were beginning to circulate in Abidjan, both in HIV prevention materials and in pornography. In the popular press, sex between men emerged as a social fact under the rubric of "homosexuality." This was helped along by the emergence of a vibrant press after the move from a one-party state in 1989. Private newspapers flourished in Abidjan, which had a literate market large enough to support them. From the mid-1990s, this press competed for readers. Rumors of homosexuality, largely concerning shadowy figures in high places and pedophilia rings, joined the staple of sensationalist stories that also addressed witchcraft, infidelities, and political corruption. They reached a crescendo by mid-1998, when some of these stories started making it into the tabloid press:

> Next August 6th, according to our indiscreet police sources, the town of Tiassalé will be the meeting point of this country's pederasts. By holding a conference there, they wish to force the authorities to legalize their relationships by drafting a law authorizing [homosexual] marriages. True or false, we'll wait and see. We'll have seen everything in this country. (*Le National*, 3 August 1998, 12)

Many of these rumors circulated outside of the printed press. They concerned political figures and constituted a vibrant political commentary. They proliferated at a time of growing national malaise. The death of President Houphouët in late 1993 was followed by the devaluation of the CFA franc, whose value was halved overnight, from fifty to the French franc to one hundred to the French franc. The devaluation was a powerful symbol of Côte-d'Ivoire's diminished standing, material proof that the crisis of the 1980s might in fact become a permanent condition. The devaluation confirmed people's fears that, without Houphouët, widely viewed as the Father of the Nation and credited for steering the nation to its economic pinnacle, they were now powerless in the face of global capitalism. The hopes and dreams nurtured during the "miracle" years appeared increasingly illusory.

Selling devaluation to the public, particularly the urban public most sensitive to its effect on the cost of living, was not an easy job. Extravagant promises were made that economic growth would result. From a macroeconomic point of view, devaluation did appear to work, rendering Ivoirian exports more competitive and kick-starting a languishing economy. But the results never materialized in everyday life, and by 1998 suspicions were high that the "devaluation dividend" had been "eaten" by those in power.[3] Rumors about predatory sexual practices by powerful men worked to extend the metaphor of illicit consumption into the more charged realm of sexuality. The World Bank's suspension of aid for "transparency concerns" in early 1999 fed these suspicions, which were confirmed later that year when the European Union also suspended aid after an audit revealed that 18 billion CFA francs (equivalent to 45 million Canadian dollars) were "missing" from the Health Ministry. As in the coverage of the "war of the sexes" that preceded it, sexuality—in this case, homosexuality—was for the press a moral barometer indexed to declining economic fortunes.

A Moral Economy of Secrecy

One of the first HIV community groups in Abidjan was Positive Nation, started in 1993. Its two founders, Christophe and Kouakou, explained to me that when they set up the organization there was little interest in the AIDS epidemic in Côte-d'Ivoire. They attributed this lack of interest to the prevailing view at the time that AIDS was "a disease of poor people, drug addicts, and Western homosexuals," and therefore not a problem in Côte-d'Ivoire. Christophe and Kouakou disagreed with this view, recounting how "many of our friends were sick or died of AIDS." Positive Nation was clearly modeled on AIDS groups in the United States and France, groups which had emerged from the gay activism of the 1970s and 1980s. Positive Nation had a flashy logo and explicitly claimed an activist stake in the fight against HIV and AIDS in Côte-d'Ivoire. Christophe showed me one of Positive Nation's colorful and slickly produced AIDS prevention pamphlets, which contained cartoon figures illustrating how to use condoms. Some of the cartoons showed two men, while others showed a man and a woman. Such a frank depiction of homosexual sex was extremely unusual in HIV prevention materials in Africa in the late 1990s. While the sexual explicitness of the educational materials was clearly inspired by posters and pamphlets the group collected from French organizations, it was also a strategy to claim a space where homosexuality could be affirmed.[4] Christophe and Kouakou themselves were homosexual. The illness and death they had witnessed involved other men who were part of what they explained to me was the "milieu." The milieu was a code word used to refer to a vaguely defined network of men who had sex with men. I got to know the milieu through my friendship with both Christophe and Kouakou.

Coverage in the popular press assumed that homosexuality was an essential attribute that defines who one is. This reflected the commonsense view of homosexuality found in France and other Western countries. This assumption also shows how talk about sex could serve as a broad commentary on how social changes affected individuals. The notion that homosexuality was an essential identity was belied by a more complicated and differentiated reality revealed through my friendship with Christophe and Kouakou. In the milieu, talk about sex circulated as secrets, and secrets were traded within discrete social networks. There, sexual secrets offered a glimpse into how talk about sex was not just a barometer of declining economic fortunes but also strategic information in the kind of battleground Vidal earlier alluded to in her description of a "war of the sexes." Sexual identity was a concept that had a specific and tactical resonance in the milieu.

While Christophe and Kouakou were quite open about being gay, this was unusual. For most in the milieu, the question of sexual identity was a vexed one. They spoke instead of having "entered" the milieu because someone "got me into it" (*On m'a mis dedans*). I had become used to hearing the phrase to denote the practice of an illicit trade. In that context, the phrase referred to the opacity of the parallel economy and the necessity of being initiated or brought "into the know" to succeed. This suggested that the self-fashioning used to master a trade described in the previous chapter might also apply to sexuality. Were these men talking about prostitution, or was something else at stake?

Many men told me they were suspicious of those they called "economic bisexuals," men who also had girlfriends and were therefore assumed to be sleeping with men for money. Yet in my conversations with bisexual men, a more ambiguous story emerged. For many, relationships with other men blended sex with longing for emotional and material comfort in ways that could not be dissociated. A relationship with a man meant being loved and taken care of in a way that was not possible with a woman, where it was expected that the man be the generous provider and source of material support. Some bisexual men had girlfriends as a "cover," while others dreamed of marrying and starting a family. It was not unusual to encounter a young man who was married with children and who continued a romantic relationship with another man, often introduced as the children's "uncle." In a setting of pervasive poverty, desire embraced economic and emotional hungering. Sexual appetites need not determine one's identity.

Most of the men I met in the milieu did not describe themselves as "homosexual" or "gay"—or even "bisexual." Euphemisms such as *branché* (trendy) were used. Sleeping with men was not something they viewed as defining who they were. For many, the secrets conveyed through rumors, gossip, and even pornography were about learning the ropes, about being part of a milieu where sex could more easily translate into love, emotional support, and even financial security. They were not revelations of a hidden identity. Rumors, gossip, and other secrets about wealthier men were treated like trade secrets, privileged insider information that could be used to gain access to a privileged club. They were valuable tools for self-fashioning in order to make oneself desirable. The cheek-by-jowl social inequality of the city meant that getting food into one's stomach, or perhaps even getting rich, was just a story away. Such stories were testimonials that could net a sugar daddy, teach a good scam, reveal a business secret, find a miraculous cure, or procure a meal. Sex talk could serve as a social technology, another tool for navigating urban life. But was it a technology of the self in the way confessional technologies and the disclosures they produced in the time of AIDS were?

I began to think so, as further conversations made me realize the complexity and gravity of being "gotten into it." "It" was a place where emotional and material longing were powerfully linked to sex, and where sexuality, rather than being a place where the truth about the self could be fixed, constituted a domain of possibility. "It" was where the regimes of discipline and training that mediated success in a parallel economy could extend to one's sexuality. However, unlike bodybuilding to obtain work as a security guard, mastering the art of persuasion to survive as a peddler, and embodying the gymnastic habitus of a skilled fare-collector, these regimes fashioned a more intimate substrate: physical desire and emotion. As in the case of the medical secret of being HIV positive, access to sexual secrets could be granted only by talking about personal experience. Anxiety about whether one's sexual longings and acts might define who one "truly" was afflicted only those who did not need to worry about survival. As in the case of an HIV diagnosis, when it came to disclosure, something more serious than reputation was at stake: survival.

Rumors were a valuable social resource that allowed men to meet each other without getting into trouble. Theft and violence were a constant fear, particularly for men who sought out encounters with rough characters. The milieu included a number of wealthy men, some of them foreigners, fuelling suspicions that "entering" could offer access to wealth and that many men engaged in homosexual behavior only for money. Much was at stake in the question of sexual identity—the question of who one really *is* sexually. For these wealthier men, someone "truly" attracted to men would not be a thief, or wouldn't engage in the dreaded but common practice of blackmail after sex, and vice versa. It was the confluence of sex, desire, and money that raised the issue of a "true" self for men whose desire led them to risk theft, beating, or blackmail. In these discussions, "true" identity was seen as a more reliable indicator of trustworthiness than homosexual behavior alone. Details about sex between men, in the milieu, took the form of secrets exchanged among conspirators, secrets whose value lay in their power to decode social relations and navigate a perilous environment. For some, these were "trade" secrets that could allow access to a better life, much in the way mastering narratives of living with HIV could broker access to life-saving drugs. For others, secrets disclosed were used to assess who could be trustworthy, much as Abdoulaye did when he brought Issa into his organization.

The milieu existed largely through a moral economy of secrecy, a community based on the exchange of valuable secrets. When a pornographic film featuring some of these men made its way back to Abidjan despite the assurances of the French producers that it would not, the moral economy was breached. Secrets—the images of the men engaging in sexual acts with other men—circulated outside the milieu. The circulation of the images made some actors into sought-after sexual commodities. Of course, the disclosure of this "secret" also had egregious consequences. Some of the actors were "outed" to family. One attempted suicide. The film's images shamed many of the actors. Their masculinity was compromised in the eyes of family because of both the behavior depicted and the assumption that they would do that for money. The circulation of the film's images outside a community bound together by a shared secret violated the moral economy. The consequences could be dramatic.

Caught in the economic vice that squeezed Côte-d'Ivoire from the 1990s, sexual and economic desire blended, making the "truth" of sexual identity increasingly difficult to locate. In the milieu, talk about sex outlined a moral economy of secrets. Secrets were traded within networks where sex and money were ambivalently linked, weapons within a battleground shaped by the "zero-sum economics" of life in a perpetual state of crisis. The prevailing national climate of suspicion linked sexual and political transgression. Under these conditions, further breaches of this moral economy could take on significance far beyond the acts of single individuals.

A National Scandal

In August 1998, *Soir-Info*, one of the Abidjan tabloid newspapers, published a *fait divers* (short news item) on its front page: "*Un libanais appréhendé pour pédophilie*" (Lebanese man arrested for pedophilia). The story concerned Monsieur Nabil, well known in the town of Dabou, sixty kilometers west of Abidjan, because he was the owner of a local watering hole called the "TGV."[5] The story reported that a local fourteen-year-old boy had accused Nabil of repeated sexual assaults, leading to his arrest. This story was not published by any of the other papers. This was not surprising, as *Soir-Info* had a reputation of trying to "use the homosexuality angle" to sell newspapers, while the others had different marketing strategies. *Soir-Info*'s sarcastic reporting of a transvestite meeting in 1994 so enraged the alleged transvestites that they descended on the newspaper's offices the next day, assaulting journalists and breaking a number of windows (Reuters, Abidjan, 14 September 14 1994). This event precipitated the formation of the Transvestites' Association (ATCI).

In what initially appeared to be an unrelated event, two weeks after Monsieur Nabil's arrest, President Bédié announced a cabinet shuffle. Seven ministers lost their portfolios, including the minister for economic infrastructure. But a week after the cabinet shuffle, *Soir-Info* reported that the affair of the "pedophile arrested in Dabou" had rebounded. Two of the presumed pedophile's brothers were arrested. The brothers were suspected of having incarcerated a young girl because she "knew too much" about their brother's activities. The story simmered on the fait divers pages of *Soir-Info* until it took a dramatic turn on 5 October 1998, a few days after the file was transmitted from the Dabou police to the Abidjan office of the Procureur de la République (District Attorney). *Le Jour*, a respectable daily and a leading opposition paper, headlined its front page with "14-year-old adolescent repeatedly sodomized; prominent figures cited" and, in subtitles "UAA, a 14-year-old youth, and pupil in a secondary school in Dabou . . . has been the victim of pedophilia on the part of a group of persons including the Minister for Economic Infrastructure, the Lebanese Ambassador, and several other prominent figures." The paper interviewed UAA and published the transcript. It details a long and lurid tale of abduction to a karaoke club in a BMW with tinted mirrors, drugging with mysterious white powders, and subsequent sexual assault.

Following the article, six of the protagonists named in the story were arrested. The mother of one of the men suffered a heart attack during the arrest and died a few days later. The paper published a certificate from a doctor certifying that the boy had been "repeatedly sodomized." Two days later the minister named in the story sued the paper for libel. The ambassador who was also implicated held a press conference pointing out that he had been out of the country the day of the alleged assault.

The affair attracted banner headlines ("Minister Declares: I am Not Homosexual"; "Pedophilia in Côte-d'Ivoire: The World Scandalized") as well as copious commentary. Parallels were drawn with Marc Dutroux, the notorious pedophile and murderer who had been arrested two years earlier in Belgium (he was convicted in 2004). In letters to the editor, "man-in-the-street" interviews, and quotes from prominent figures, Ivoirians expressed their horror. Many noted that this was contrary to African traditions, a sign of moral decay, and that decadent foreigners clearly felt license to do as they wished in Côte-d'Ivoire.

The affair was also political. The ruling party closed ranks around the accused minister, supporting his libel suit, and argued that the accusations were a political dirty trick. Opposition papers played up the affair. Friends told me "Let's not forget this is all happening under the Bédié régime." Delegations from political parties and youth groups visited the "young sodomite" to express their moral support. One observer noted that this "is not just a banal homosexual incident" and that "homosexuality and lesbianism have rotted the social body to the point where organizations like the Transvestites' Association of Côte-d'Ivoire can set up shop unopposed." The affair dragged on for the rest of the year, with the minister finally winning his libel suit against the newspaper. The six men who had been arrested were eventually released. One of them later died from illness contracted while in jail.

While the *affaire pédophilie* may have given voice to the widespread dissatisfaction, even disgust, with the Bédié régime, it also demonstrated how "sexual deviance" was a powerful metaphor for expressing concerns about the republic. By the mid-1990s, the country appeared to be in a terminal economic decline that had begun with the collapse of the "Ivoirian" miracle of the 1970s. In the deepening economic gloom, this decline was attributed to corruption, and political figures were suspected of harboring secret wealth and other ill-gotten gains. As the First Republic unraveled in the late 1990s after the death of Houphouët, rumors of corruption and nepotism spread. Scandal—more precisely, the unveiling of scandalous secrets—became the idiom for expressing anxieties about the state of the nation and the vulnerability of its citizens. The ease with which the pedophilia affair became a media sensation echoed how sex had served as a moral barometer in the 1970s. Transformed economic and political fortunes had, however, reframed moral questions in terms of decline rather than "modernization."

Suspicions and Fears

UAA, it turned out, was known within the milieu as a "twisted little queen," a manipulative character "not to be trusted" and who was not a minor. Many told me they suspected that he was being manipulated by political forces and perhaps even being paid off. Such observations reflected the perception that UAA had in fact betrayed others with whom he shared the secret of his homosexual activities. The death in jail of one of those charged in the scandal shook the milieu where he was well known. For a while nightclubs were shunned, as many feared a witch hunt. "It doesn't take much to stir things up around here," I was frequently told. One prominent feminist activist I interviewed, who had been particularly outspoken in denouncing an "epidemic" of sexual abuse in Ivoirian families, told me that she felt there was something "not straight" about UAA when he came to seek her support for his case. "He wouldn't look me in the eye," she noted. After my investigations, I was left with the nagging suspicion that UAA's narrative was just a piece of gossip that had somehow gotten out of hand. UAA's unreliability was easy enough to determine. So why did Le Jour publish such an outlandish story? The editor explained to me that "we had to" since the initial arrest of Monsieur Nabil was public record, as were the subsequent explosive declarations accusing public figures of being in the sex ring.

I eventually tracked UAA down but never got the chance to interview him. The rumor network of the milieu had located him in an anonymous section of one of the newer townships, where the roads were not yet paved and impromptu housing filled in the space between half-finished apartment blocks. UAA had taken to wearing obviously effeminate clothing, I was told: flared Capri pants, slip-on wedgies, and even once, a simple *pagne* (lappa cloth) wrapped around the waist. In the neighborhood he was a curiosity and a source of gossip. My contact did not want to have anything to do with him, precluding any chance of an introduction. "People say he's just like that . . . but I don't want people thinking *I'm* like that," my contact concluded firmly. The visibility of UAA's sexual identity and the way it anchored gossip in the neighborhood threatened to contaminate the reputation of those who associated with him. So why were his accusations so potent?

In Côte-d'Ivoire's never-ending economic crisis, wealth, it was assumed, came from theft: a zero-sum economy. Many Ivoirians told me that politicians, who never seemed to suffer from the deteriorating economic conditions, were "eating our money." Suspicions of political-economic transgression were confirmed with the suspension of aid from donors such as the World Bank and the European Union in 1999. The inkling that corruption, as evidence of the political and moral decay of the nation, must be linked to other, unspeakable acts was given voice by UAA's disclosures. In the climate of suspicion that reigned in Abidjan in the late 1990s, public disclosures such as UAA's breached a moral economy of secrecy but gained a wider currency as a moral barometer. By bringing to light what everyone suspected was happening behind the scenes, his disclosure was a broad accusation. It foreshadowed what, at the time, was an unthinkable dénouement to the political anxieties raised by the scandal.

Fall of the First Republic

In 1999 Christmas Eve fell on a Friday, the last working day before a long weekend. As nearly half of Abidjanais are Muslim, many leave work early for Friday prayers. That day rush hour began at noon. I was working at the clinic, where we were writing up the last round of lab results, when cell phones began to ring simultaneously. Reports came in of an armed robbery at the Sococe shopping center in the wealthy suburb of 2-Plateaux, perpetrated by bandits dressed as soldiers. Over the next hours, more cell-phone reports flowed in of the robbery and of mysterious troop movements throughout the capital. The central business district of the Plateau had already begun to empty out for the long weekend when the reports started, and the pace accelerated as the last office workers scurried home, worried about getting stuck in traffic. By then there was a palpable sense that something was amiss. Where we were in Zone four, one bridge away from the Plateau to the north—and another bridge again from 2-Plateaux—everything was calm, but the reports of soldiers moving around and massing in the Plateau seemed out of the ordinary.

As the reports proliferated and soldiers were spotted as far away as Yopougon, far to the west, and then at the international airport to the east, people started tuning in to Radio France International (RFI) to get the latest news. By the time I had walked from the clinic to my friend Abass's apartment not far away, RFI had managed to interview soldiers who claimed to be mutineering over back pay they claimed they were owed from a UN peacekeeping mission in the Central African Republic. That night, most people stayed in, and I stayed at Abass's. Something seemed not quite right. I called a friend in Montréal and told him what was going on—about the soldiers that had popped up all around the city, at the airport, and the radio and television stations. "Sounds like a coup," he said. It was unthinkable. Côte-d'Ivoire had never had a coup and indeed had been a bastion of political stability ever since independence, even throughout the economic crisis of the 1980s and the tumultuous transition to multiparty democracy in the 1990s.

The next morning, General Robert Gueï spoke on national radio and television, announcing that President Bédié, the head of state, had been deposed, the institutions of the First Republic were henceforth suspended by the Committee of National Salvation, of which General Gueï was the head, and that a state of emergency had been declared. It *was* a coup. Gueï spoke of the need to clean house and heal a diseased republic. Many Ivoirians shared this sentiment. They were tired of the proliferating scandals and widespread corruption that they felt characterized Bédié's regime and suspicious of Bédié's attempts to marginalize his main political opponents, namely the former prime minister Alassane Dramane Ouattara. I ventured out to meet Yao in Treichville. There was no public transportation, and I didn't see any cabs, so I resolved to walk the four kilometers to Treichville. It was a foolish move. I was almost killed twice that day, once by a wildly swerving jeep full of cheering supporters and, much later, when a drunken soldier shot at us. Still, it allowed me to witness the energies and the violence that a political void, however brief, may unleash.

By the time I met up with Yao in Treichville, crowds had gathered in the streets, cheering whenever they saw soldiers. The crowds were jubilant, the mood optimistic. Yao and I made our way to the Plateau, crossing the Charles de Gaulle Bridge with a stream of other pedestrians. Yao had purchased a goat for Christmas from a merchant north of the Plateau in Dokui and had resolved to get it by hook or by crook. Here and there, we saw vehicles that had been abandoned on the side of the road, having run out of petrol, as gas stations had all closed. We talked to people along the way, and, several hours later, we started coming across the first inmates who had been released from the Maison d'Arrêt et de Correction d'Abidjan (MACA), the overcrowded and foreboding prison that lay a few hours on foot to the west. By then plumes of smoke were rising from all four quarters of the city and the mood had become apprehensive. Somehow, it had dawned on people that it wasn't clear what was going to happen. Bédié had still neither been seen nor heard.

Yao and I had stopped at a roadside stall to drink when RFI reported that the French Socialist prime minister, Lionel Jospin, had said that France would stand by and not take sides. France maintained an important military base beside the airport, and in the past had consistently intervened to prop up imperiled leaders in its former African colonies. "Bédié's finished," said one young woman sitting around the stall as she braided a friend's hair. Prime Minister Jospin had been quick to state France's position himself in order to pre-empt President Chirac, whom he feared might choose another course since he belonged to a rightist party. France's awkward "cohabitation" between a president and prime minister of opposing parties injected an element of uncertainty into the Ivoirian crisis. A few minutes later, RFI controversially broadcast an interview with Bédié, who spoke in his unmistakable voice. Its resemblance to the drawl of his predecessor, Côte-d'Ivoire's first president and Father of the Nation Félix Houphouët-Boigny, had long nurtured suspicions that Bédié was an illegitimate son of Houphouët's. He called emphatically for the "forces of the republic" to "actively resist" this usurpation of power. His lilt echoed that of Houphouët, who had been dead for six years. It made it seem eerily like Houphouët was speaking from the grave.

The mood changed instantly. After we obtained the goat and met up with some other friends, we made our way back to Zone four. We found a taxi to take us, with the unfortunate beast bundled into the trunk. I can still remember its hoofs kicking me through the paper-thin back seat. When we got to the Charles de Gaulle Bridge, a roadblock had been set up using a burnt-out bus laid perpendicular to traffic. The heavily armed rebel soldiers manning the roadblock motioned to me to get out. Despite French Prime Minister Jospin's announcement, they were nervous, expecting the French to intervene at any moment. They were agitated, but in the end they let us go once they saw my Canadian passport and heard that I was a doctor. By then, looting had started. We rode through a deserted Zone four, swerving to avoid debris scattered over the roadway. The tallest building in the quarter, the ten-story headquarters of Ivoiris, a French-owned cell-phone company, was in flames. It has been torched by rebel sympathizers who blamed France for supporting Bédié and wanted to send a clear message that French interference was not welcome. That night we could hear music mixed with gunfire as soldiers, many of them drunk, celebrated their victory.

The Second Republic

General Gueï lasted only ten months. He was assassinated after he tried to steal the election that brought President Laurent Gbagbo to power in late 2000. Gbagbo pursued Bédié's policy of *Ivoirité* (Ivoirianness), which linked national identity to specific ethnic groups. Bédié's policy had been used to disqualify his principal political rival, the former prime minister Alassane Dramane Ouattara. Gbagbo argued that Ouattara was not truly Ivoirian since he was born in northern Côte-d'Ivoire. This area is heavily populated by ethnic groups with roots in neighboring countries. That Ouattara was also a rival of Gbagbo's may have explained why the new president saw political advantage in extending his predecessor's policy. Ironically, Ivoirité was built on the ethnic divisions created by French colonial policies of classification. In this case, colonial dividing practices were still visible in Ivoirité's ethnic cartography, which provided a grid of intelligibility for enacting a political triage to separate those who could legitimately aspire to power from those who could not.

Many blamed the policy of Ivoirité for an even more dramatic insurrection two years into Gbagbo's term. In 2002 rebel forces shelled Abidjan in an attempt to oust him from office. Northerners who resented the attempt to exclude them from political participation on the basis of their assumed ethnic non-Ivoirianness led the attempt to overthrow Gbagbo. France intervened to quell the violence, fearing that the bombing and the potential for all-out civil war would lead to massive civilian casualties in a city where tens of thousands of French citizens still lived. The conflict smoldered on for five years, eventually flaring into a full-fledged civil war that partitioned the country into the rebel-held North and government-controlled South. France initially established and manned a buffer zone between the warring sides. Later on, a multinational UN stabilization force secured the buffer zone.

A fog of war enveloped the country. Rumors of plots and counterplots proliferated. Interminable "inter-Ivoirian" dialogues and reconciliation conferences ended in stalemate or agreements that were never applied.

Many Ivoirians accused the French of supporting the Northerners. In 2003 demonstrations, looting, and violence targeted the French. French schools and France's Cultural Center were ransacked. France intervened once again, sending its military to "secure" Abidjan in order to allow a mass evacuation of thousands of French citizens by a small fleet of Air France jumbo jets. French military forces set up roadblocks and in one incident fired on demonstrators, killing nearly one hundred. Ivoirian militia and death squads were suspected in the proliferation of massacres, mysterious disappearances, and deaths. The bodies of those executed washed up on the shores of the lagoons that ring Abidjan's *presqu'îles* and peninsulas. References were made to ethnic cleansing. The grid of political legibility blurred. Even at the time of this writing in 2009, with a peace accord in place, the leader of the rebel *Forces Nouvelles* (New Forces) now holding the office of prime minister, and rival militias and death squads being disarmed, the outcome remains uncertain. Presidential elections have still not been held. The country remains in a political state of suspension.

In retrospect, it seems the declining economic conditions that had increasingly come to characterize the impact of globalization on Côte-d'Ivoire fatally undermined the First Republic under Bédié and set the stage for the general's "house cleaning" on Christmas Eve of 1999. After the fall of the First Republic, colonial ethnic categories came back to haunt the Second Republic that replaced it, drawing the battle lines of Côte-d'Ivoire's civil war. The violence of the civil war hewed to the cleavages generated by colonial practices of ethnic differentiation. It unraveled the forms of national solidarity forged by Houphouet, whose rise to power was ironically enabled by the emergence of the Baoulé as a dominant ethnicity. French military interventions further undermined the sense of national sovereignty. Despite its ethnic overtones, the civil war's roots lay in the economic crisis and the struggle over resources that ensued.[6]

The economic crisis of the 1970s had produced fissures that led to new tactical innovations and forms of self-fashioning. As we saw in the previous chapter, specific forms of identity became available through practices for sorting people and were made "real" as they were taken to pragmatic ends. In the parallel economies that emerged in the wake of the economic crisis, the ability to transform one's self became valuable. Bodybuilders became night watchmen and a security industry thrived; youth trained to become fare collectors or hucksters. This continued through the civil unrest, as Dozo warriors—youth clad in traditional dress and rumored to be immune to patrolled neighborhoods and were sought out as security guards.[7]

Concluding Remarks: Making up People

Through the story of homosexuality and politics during the time of AIDS, we have seen how disclosure in the milieu's moral economy of secrecy adhered to a logic that located the truth of "sexuality" deep in the self and, more broadly, assigned truth to secrets revealed. "Sex" could serve as a moral barometer, as a way of telling the "truth" about social and political transformation.[8] Two overlapping régimes laid claim to establishing the "truth" of disclosure: a confessional one that required that attention be directed inward, and one of accusation that focused scrutiny away from the discloser and onto the powerful. The confessional régime promoted the disclosure of secrets in a moral economy of solidarity, recalling the type of personal disclosure encouraged in the fight against AIDS. For the gay men I befriended in the milieu, the "truth" of sex was to be found be examining one's desires and the sense of self they helped shape. To disclose that knowledge of the self was to broker entry into a community of others who shared the same knowledge. In contrast, the political economy of inequality and the division it brewed anchored a régime of accusation visible in the suspicions that could greet HIV testimonials and the schisms that wracked HIV groups. The toxic political environment that characterized the last year of the First Republic led UAA's disclosures to direct attention outward. They were accusations levied at the powerful. They were the first symptoms of the political violence that would be unleashed in the wake of the fall of the First Republic.

Thus, disclosure can cut both ways: it can create social ties or, alternatively, it can dissolve social bonds. Let's recall Issa's, Jeanne's, and Matthieu's public testimonials discussed earlier in the book. These were understood as conveying the "truth" about the teller. Disclosures were encouraged with the belief that one could obtain therapeutic relief through sharing painful secrets (such as suffering from a fatal and sexually transmitted disease). Solidarity among sufferers would allegedly result in the recognition of a shared inner experience: "I feel that way too." This was the measure of the "truth" of shared disclosure. It occurred in an economy of alleged empathy and affect. Returning to the examples in chapter 1, Abdoulaye's growing doubts about Issa's testimonial of being HIV positive and his certainty that Matthieu was lying to seek material gain from his testimonial, despite the proof of his HIV positivity, reflected a logic of interpretation based on this economy of empathy and affect. In contrast, the suspicion that greeted Jeanne's first HIV testimonials described in chapter 1 was borne out by the triage that enabled confessors to receive antiretrovirals, which we saw later in chapter 4. Disclosing HIV-positive status does not spontaneously result in solidarity and belonging; indeed, it can be viewed as self-serving. Disclosure can be seen as an oblique accusation directed at those with whom one would normally share such secrets: family, lovers, or friends. It can be seen as a public airing of dirty laundry. What are the implications of encouraging people to disclose in the fight against HIV? Will the results usher in new forms of solidarity as originally hoped? Or might they, in contrast, be greeted with distrust or as a form of betrayal, introducing new cleavages?

The fall of the First Republic shows the violence that may result from apparently innocuous social divisions. The dividing practices introduced by colonialism to better manage the population and the economy transformed arbitrary distinctions into real differences between people that continue to shape political struggle up to the present day. They came back to haunt Côte-d'Ivoire in the civil war. Similarly, practices of self-transformation also create differences, visible in efforts to respond to the AIDS epidemic and in the urban trades explored in the previous chapter. Technologies of the self mobilized the mysterious substance of the self into an "identity." Compromised national sovereignty, the violence of the coup, and its aftermath of civil war vividly illustrate the power of technologies of the self, evidenced by the way that "street warriors" of Abidjan's youth culture became newly agential in this context. Earlier practices of triage and disclosure generated new forms of violence.

WHO LIVES? WHO DIES?

The Politics of Triage

Triage in the time of AIDS emerges against the contours of what can be called, at least rhetorically, a long war that fashioned tactical forms of citizenship. This long war began with colonial conquest and continued, sublimated in the confrontations, negotiations, and tactical engagements with colonial rule. In French Africa the colonial state's successive attempts to grapple with "the native question" in both political and biological terms solidified social and ethnic cleavages. These were briefly forgotten with the foundation of Côte-d'Ivoire's First Republic in 1961. After independence, economic shocks and social restructuring shaped a political struggle that took an increasingly violent turn in the civil war that erupted in 2002, three years after the fall of the First Republic in 1999. Colonial cleavages returned to haunt the Second Republic that ensued.

In the time of AIDS in Côte-d'Ivoire, a ruined economy and a "zero-sum" cultural logic were the background against which practices of selection became intertwined with narrative techniques by which the truth of selves could be told. Mastery counted: talking about yourself came to be about getting ARV drugs and staying alive. Triage involved struggles over resources and power, delineating a fissured space of political action. Beneath the veneer of "criteria," "procedures," and a glossy rhetoric about "saving lives," in the end, it is finally about who lives and who dies and how these decisions are made: triage is not just political, it is politics.[1] More fundamentally, triage is about *sovereignty,* as the German philosopher Carl Schmitt (2005, 5) affirmed: "Sovereign is he who decides upon the exception." Since the first efforts to organize communities with HIV in West Africa in 1994, this has become increasingly clear.

Triage is a technology of exception, deployed in the context of emergency. It separates who must live from who may die. It is a mobile and partial exercise of therapeutic sovereignty. In its early and untamed form, as examples in chapter 4 show, it was unnoticed because it was ignored: it raised too many uncomfortable questions. As triage becomes institutionalized, it remains largely invisible because we only count those who are saved: those who are enrolled into programs deployed within an evidence-generating machine. Difficult decisions to ration scarce resources are, of course, made everywhere. In wealthy countries, triage is a comparatively transparent political process, visible in debates over waiting times, treatment priorities, insurance coverage, and the way health budgets are allocated. Debates over Canada's lower rates of cardiac surgery relative to the United States or the difficulty of obtaining dialysis for the elderly in Britain are examples of open discussions that ensue when health care is rationed.

This ethnographic exploration of efforts to combat AIDS in French West Africa has shown how triage escaped the control of a usually rational political institution such as the state as national sovereignty eroded. It resulted from technologies of the self "gone rogue." Triage in the time of AIDS is a virulent mutant of earlier forms of colonial and postcolonial discrimination. It is a recombinant in which colonial and postcolonial technologies of exclusion are visible. These include colonial technologies that segregated "natives" in the name of hygiene and to safeguard settler health; technologies of difference that mapped ethnicity; and postcolonial technologies of government that ruled through selectively destroying habitations. Neoliberal technologies of "structural adjustment" transformed economic inequality into a zero-sum game. In opposition, tactical innovations were deployed. These included forms of discipline and technologies of the self.

This new form of triage is highly virulent because it produces physical exclusion, economic inequality, and even highly graduated biological differences within social groups. Differences in access to therapy have affected immune systems and viral resistance patterns. Subtle biological gradations have formed between individuals who have had access to more or better drugs and those who have had less. Bodies are infected by an HIV that is now drug-resistant and are marked by toxic ARV drugs such as d4T that are shunned in wealthy countries. Triage is corrosive to social ties. It introduces mechanisms of selection that inadvertently pit people against one another. In matters of life and death, it confronts newer forms of biomedical belonging that promise treatment with existing social ties based on reciprocity. Triage forced Abdoulaye and others profiled in this book to negotiate conflicting moral economies, and led to fission and competition within and among self-help groups.

Therapeutic Citizenship or Biotribalism?

What kind of struggle may be possible in this situation? Therapeutic citizenship is more than a metaphor. As delivery systems for drugs are ramped up, they increasingly become a conduit for a host of other services. In Burkina Faso and Côte-d'Ivoire and in other African nations, I have seen how drugs and counseling may now come bundled with food aid, microcredit, school fees for orphans and vulnerable children, and more. This ever-growing package of services calls forth an ever-more complex assemblage of institutions and management systems, an alphabet soup of acronyms and programs that make a rendering of accountability virtually impossible. Yet for many beneficiaries of these programs, these may be the only meaningful forms of material citizenship to which they have access. Paradoxically this situation reiterates the way most Africans in the colonial period first acceded to citizenship as biological objects of colonial public health programs, bodies for labor in the colonial economy, or subjects of taxation. Citizenship in our postcolonial age seems to be granted in these cases on the basis of a disease, to victims in need of saving. A form of value emerges from the statistics of an AIDS industry that counts bodies treated and lives saved.

There are two ways to read this situation. We have seen the divisive potential of treatment programs. These mobilize new forms of biopolitical triage to shower resources on the "lucky" few. These programs are eerily reminiscent of early colonial policies of ethnic differentiation that in Côte-d'Ivoire drew the fault lines of current conflicts. A pessimistic reading would then see in the rise of therapeutic citizenship the potential for therapeutic colonization and a slow progression toward biotribalism that could sow the seeds of future conflicts. This could even lead to "iatrogenic violence" (McFalls 2007) as people "refuse" treatment through whatever means available.[2]

Alternatively, from these many years of engagement with people affected by HIV in Africa, it is possible to see in therapeutic citizenship the rudiments of a new form of "biosociality" (Rabinow 1992). This suggests the possibility that a shared biological condition may foster new forms of belonging, however fragile. Over the years, I have seen how the treatments return people to health. Abdoulaye, like many members of the HIV groups I have worked with, sought a partner who was already HIV positive, so as not to risk transmitting the infection. He and others explained to me that, now that they were healthy, they wanted to continue with their lives and start families. They married and, knowing that the treatments would practically eliminate the risk of transmitting HIV to offspring, bore children. In the past five years, several of the members of the groups I worked with have had healthy children.

An examination of colonial history reveals parallels with community HIV groups like Jeunes sans frontières. Like the many voluntary associations that preceded them, these groups express the aspirations—the desire for progress, self-fashioning, and mastery in a social world fraught with contingency—by which Africans have, since the colonial era, sought to orient their entry into the global order. Current mobilization around the issue of access to treatment bears witness to the ability of tactics fashioned on the peripheries of the world system to leverage social change with global implications. Far from being a story of despair and hopelessness—merely another trope of the "coming anarchy" arguments that rehearse self-serving ideas of Africa as a perpetual heart of darkness—these stories point to the potential, even the necessity, of progress against all odds.

Body Counts

At a meeting in London in 1998, I recall a senior French official berating an epidemiologist who had conducted the first AZT trials for prevention of mother-to-child transmission of HIV in West Africa, described in chapter 4. "I need to treat three thousand women, and you can't come up with them?" he complained. In order to govern a population by an exceptional AIDS response, that population must first exist and be available, which is not the case when the vast majority of the potentially HIV-positive population has minimal access to health care, let alone HIV testing. That population must therefore be called into being through procedures that allow it to be identified, separated from those who are not subject to intervention, *and* counted—in other words, a systematic triage. The need to quantify and assemble evidence that results have been achieved drives a powerful metrics of rescue.

By 2003, massive financial commitments to pay for antiretroviral drugs in developing countries had been made by the newly established Global Fund for AIDS, Tuberculosis, and Malaria, and the United States' President's Emergency Program for AIDS Relief (PEPFAR), initiated by then-president George W. Bush.[3] As these words are being written (December 2009), the total number of people receiving antiretroviral therapy (ART) through humanitarian mass HIV treatment programs is estimated at slightly over 3 million (UNAIDS 2008). The Global Fund and PEPFAR each claim they are treating around two million, reflecting significant "double counting" of patients treated in sites that are jointly funded, as well as the need to show results in terms of "numbers of lives saved" (PEPFAR 2009, 15). By the end of 2008, PEPFAR estimated it was treating upwards of fifty thousand in Côte-d'Ivoire alone.[4]

Mass treatment programs require "body counts" (see H. Epstein 2008, 213–28) of people on treatment and even of their physical condition. This evidence is a lubricant for keeping resources flowing from program funders, who must prove to their constituents that their money is being used to achieve stated ends. For instance, both PEPFAR and the Global Fund measure and report "numbers of lives saved" and "years of lives saved" (3.28 million estimated for PEPFAR to September 2009, PEPFAR 2009, 7) to prove their effectiveness. Without a population to rescue, however, programs cannot generate the desired outcomes, much less evidence that results are being achieved.

The recent change in the collection and analysis of HIV statistics based on surveillance of specific groups reveals the science of this systematic triage. Earlier methods used estimates drawn from studies of high-risk populations (pregnant women, those with sexually transmitted infections or TB, and hospitalized patients), a group that is readily available through the health care system. Starting in the early 2000s, these were gradually being replaced by random household surveys, which are a much more accurate reflection of the population rates.[5] This shift makes sense in the context of a program that aggressively seeks to map the population available through more accurate measuring. This may then firmly establish a narrow "denominator" against which the success of enrollment efforts can be measured, while excluding those who are not eligible for intervention.

Proving that lives are being saved requires more than just instituting a body count of patients on antiretrovirals. Patients must also be monitored for lengths of time sufficient to observe and record therapeutic effects of the drugs (at minimum a year). This is also a challenge, particularly where the technology to identify and monitor the population is absent or functions poorly and where identity documents are unreliable, often obtained multiple times from different sources and of poor quality. Indeed, counterfeits are often better made than official documents, as described in chapter 4. For instance, from interviews I conducted in Côte-d'Ivoire in late 2007, I learned that PEPFAR had developed a sophisticated software program to track both monies and people as they converge for treatment; in Zambia "smart cards" are being used to monitor patients (PEPFAR 2007, 159; see Amoore 2006 for a general discussion of "biometric borders"). Recently, evidence that significant numbers of patients drop out of treatment programs has caused alarm. "Loss to follow-up," as this is termed, is of some concern as it means that the virus of patients who go off their drugs or are not strictly adherent may develop resistance and be spread—an issue certain to spur the development of more sophisticated strategies to track and monitor patients.

Getting body counts therefore requires that people be identified and grouped so that they may be enrolled into an apparatus where they can be subject to intervention and the results quantified. Enrollment may generate evidence, but it may also produce new social relations between those enrolled. Confessional technologies employed to encourage testing (chapter 2) or recruitment of women into AZT trials in West Africa (chapter 4) helped bring about a therapeutic citizenship. The lives of those who are not enrolled into these interventions, those who, in the words of the informant I cited in chapter 4, have been "discarded," no longer count. Triage identifies those whose lives are to be saved and counted; but what of those left by the wayside?

A Broader Triage

For the millions living with HIV who are now on lifesaving drugs and for those who can no longer stand by helplessly, the rise of mass HIV treatment programs is something to be celebrated. However, a brief idyll of therapeutic optimism has recently been punctured by the sobering realities of delivering the drugs in a landscape littered with the wreckage of health systems barely able to deliver basic services. It is in that landscape that the governments of wealthy Northern countries and high-powered NGOs intervene, followed by an armada of smaller organizations borne by a tide of funding. The AIDS programs of large countries such as the United States or France now jockey for position, rivaled by private philanthropies such as the Gates Foundation, private-public partnerships such as the Global Fund for AIDS, Tuberculosis, and Malaria, or even multinational corporations' AIDS relief programs. Laurie Garrett (2007) has argued that these well-funded global actors are in some places cannibalizing what little public infrastructure is left as they lure doctors and nurses into AIDS programs with higher salaries. AIDS drugs and programs compete for hearts and minds—and bodies. When activists told me of bidding wars to entice patients to enroll in treatment programs, I remembered how prophets fought over converts in colonial Côte-d'Ivoire. Little is left for those who suffer from other diseases. Reporting on an extensive ethnography of health among the urban poor in Delhi, Veena Das and Ranendra Das share a similar reflection as they consider the death, from tuberculosis, of a young woman. They note that the "'letting die' happens even as international agencies and the government participate in the global Stop TB program . . . terms such as *abandonment* or *triage* cannot be deployed in a seamless manner as we traverse the milieu of the family and the state" (Das and Das 2007, 86–87).

On a recent trip to Abidjan, I spent a day with a close friend. While I was with him, he kept getting phone calls that he would answer in an urgent, impatient, and pleading voice that I was not used to hearing him use. After the fourth call, I indiscreetly asked, "What's the matter?" "It's Kouassi," he told me, "he needs money again." "For what?" "His dialysis." Kouassi, whom I had met many years earlier, had recently been diagnosed with kidney failure at age twenty-eight—not an uncommon condition in developing countries, where infections and toxins can imperceptibly damage kidneys until they no longer work. A kidney transplant was out of the question and only expensive dialysis kept him alive. His family and friends financially exhausted, Kouassi died two weeks later.

Mass HIV interventions have taken triage to a whole new level, as they select out people with HIV for lifesaving treatment while others who also face illness and even death from non-HIV diseases are left behind. Flows of money for HIV treatment do not occur in isolation. They are a small part of global resource flows, such as those for development aid, debt relief, trade subsidies, and the purchase of goods and services that determine how much can be spent on health in general.[6] These capital flows enact a more general triage, whereby the selection of those with HIV who should receive drugs has been displaced by a selection of diseases that merit treatment. We live in a world where, for millions, death stalks every fever, every pregnancy, and even minor injuries. Paradoxically, as mass HIV treatment programs cleave those who benefit from those who do not, this may become a world where some-times the only way to survive is by having a fatal illness called HIV.

An Uncertain Future

That HIV has now become a mainstream issue clearly represents a victory over the hesitations and equivocations of an international aid industry that all too often lost track of the people it was trying to help, as Madame Janvier at the World Bank admitted. Yet even as the drugs are pumped into Africa and other poor countries, doubts remain about the adequacy of the response. The epi-demic continues to spread. Not enough people are receiving treatment. The expanded use of antiretrovirals reveals the glaring inability of a weakened health system to manage. There are not enough trained people to handle the drugs, even as desperate program managers use higher salaries to poach staff from general health care institutions. Growing biological resistance to the drugs has recently emerged as an issue, fuelled by drug stock-outs and insuf-ficient resources to properly monitor therapy.

As mass HIV treatment programs enroll millions, they are confronted not only with the challenge of ensuring adherence to treatment but also with the paradoxical effects of treatment. My clinical experience in Canada had taught me that antiretroviral treatment increases patients' appetites. But when ac-cess to food is limited, as was the case in the groups I followed, as patients got better, they grew hungrier. Working with people enrolled in treatment pro-grams in Mozambique, medical anthropologist Ippolytos Kalofonos (2008) has explored the consequences of this previously unremarked effect of treat-ment, which prompted some to complain that all they eat are ARVs. Yet pro-viding food to people on treatment as entire communities go hungry gen-erates resentment and bitterness—and even a form of paranoia as people wonder who is getting what and imagine that others are eating while they go hungry. Kalofonos noted "how difficult it is that each household, regardless of the number of HIV-positive members, only receives food supplements for one individual," as he explained to me one informant's observation that "each person is eating the blood of the other."[7]

I often hear the commentary that AIDS has become a business and those who have lucked into the "business" grow plump while those who have not grow thin. In Ouagadougou, the National AIDS Committee is now housed in a shiny new office building that locals refer to as the "SIDA Business Center." The linguistic switch between the French acronym for AIDS—SIDA—and English is telling. For many I speak to, the swelling waistlines of AIDS bureaucrats confirm the suspicion that those who fatten as others struggle to survive must eat more than medicines. The prominent brand names that are lavishly displayed on the bags of USAID corn-soy blend or Canada bulgur wheat that are distributed along with antiretroviral drugs are poignant evidence that AIDS relief subtly commodifies the lives of those who suffer. Those who receive them complain that the packages are just barely enough to keep them alive. In exchange, donors cite self-congratulatory statistics (Richey 2008).

Over the past five years, I have spoken to many people in Burkina Faso, Côte-d'Ivoire, and Mali who now live healthy and productive lives thanks to the antiretrovirals. They worry that the tide of AIDS relief efforts will recede and that they will once again be "discarded." What will likely remain is a therapeutic archipelago for the lucky few and not much in between. As the realization dawns that it will not be possible, as Kevin de Cock, the head of the WHO's HIV division frequently says, to "treat our way out of the epidemic," the rather thornier problem of the lack of public health infrastructure in these territories of intervention is increasingly debated, leaving open the possibility that emergency will give way to long-term reconstruction. Will HIV programs shed the logic of fragmenting, targeting, and managing specific populations? How to translate early therapeutic success for HIV into meaningful long-term investments in public health?

A Fog of War

A fog of war has enveloped the struggle against AIDS. Former adversaries have become allies, and former allies have been torn apart—perhaps most visibly in South Africa where antiapartheid activists fell out over the ANC government's approach to the epidemic after 2000. But more importantly, tactical advantage is almost impossible to grasp on a slippery terrain where every advance is compromised by the broader war being waged all around. Mass treatment programs can work but only if they cannibalize existing health systems. Prevention programs suffer as resources shift to treatment. And the more successful the treatment program, the more work it generates for itself as the pool of patients grows through the survival of those treated and the arrival of new patients drawn by the program's success.

Some activists I have spoken to recently are disconcerted that they now find themselves on the side of the rich and powerful. "What, exactly, is the struggle against?" they ask. For a time, the fight with the pharmaceuticals industry over patent laws focused the struggle, and an easy alliance seemed possible with other antiglobalization movements. But now the drugs are flowing, Bill Gates and Bill Clinton are celebrated as the new heroes of AIDS activism, and Paul Farmer is touted as the possible new head of USAID. Yao, the activist behind the group Positive Nation, profiled in chapter 3, is now a professional AIDS manager. He traveled to Washington in late 2006 to meet then-U.S. president George W. Bush. In the official White House photographs, he is seen shaking hands with Bush, as Karl Rove, Bush's political mastermind, stands in the background. The United States Embassy in Abidjan initially denied Yao a visa to travel to the United States because he was HIV positive. The embassy relented when the White House intervened. Abdoulaye, the founder of Jeunes sans frontières, has grown it into a large organization. The Friendship Center is now a three-story building built with British and Dutch funds, where over a thousand people receive treatment for HIV. But in September 2009, the center was badly damaged by floods that struck Ouagadougou after torrential downpours. Abdoulaye's fears that his daughter Sali might be HIV positive were belied by her good health. She now has a younger sister, whom Abdoulaye fathered with his new HIV-positive girlfriend. Both children are healthy and on the verge of adolescence. Theresa, the facilitator of the confessional workshop described in chapter 2, continues to do consulting, now mainly for the UN.

In reference to Iraq, journalist Roger Cohen (2006) wrote, "war spews words." AIDS has been no exception. The proliferation of words about AIDS, from academic studies to media coverage and the saturation of public service announcements, rehearses the familiar oppositional tropes of victims and heroes, vulnerability and empowerment, illness and redemption, and balances the fiery rhetoric of activists with the cool language of outcomes, measures, and programs. I have tried to look beyond this war of words to examine the material practices that the fight against AIDS has generated. AIDS is a matter of life and death for millions. As such it has created spaces where exceptional people, like many I describe in this book, have tried to wrest control over their destinies and foster a new solidarity. But these spaces knew constraint: a logic that values some lives over others. In these spaces the poverty of the ill confronted the relative wealth of others who sought to help. The struggle to survive converged with others' need to save lives. This therapeutic alliance was constrained at every turn. There wasn't enough room on the life-boat afforded by antiretroviral therapy. The result was the gradual assemblage of mechanisms of triage and exclusion.

Government-by-Exception

Recall how in 2000, lack of access to HIV treatment suddenly became a global humanitarian emergency. The right to treatment became orthodoxy in the global health community, even for international organizations and donors that had previously argued against using HIV drugs in developing countries. A humanitarian juggernaut swept away arguments that treatment would be unaffordable, would take scarce resources from prevention programs, and could not be effectively delivered by struggling health systems. A new front was opened up in the "war on AIDS," to which a new generation of organizations flocked, ready to take up battle.

The geographical logic of these programs bears a striking resemblance to the way European powers divided up Africa in the late nineteenth century. The "scramble for Africa" and the colonial regime it installed to rule over territories and the peoples they contained resulted in arbitrary borders and ethnic cleavages that persist to this day, at times with tragic consequences (Mamdani 1996; Pakenham 1992). HIV programs do not create new borders, but they reflect a geopolitical logic in deciding who gets to intervene and where, and in doing so they produce arbitrary social borders.

France has been a pioneer of advocating access to treatment since President Chirac denounced the unavailability of ARVs in the South at the Abidjan AIDS conference in 1997 and introduced a program to have French hospitals spearhead "technical cooperation" with African counterparts. In the years following this book's accounts, I witnessed a curious result: Parisian hospitals were attributed therapeutic territories, corresponding to former French colonies, where they were to establish treatment programs. This therapeutic recolonization included hospitals in the French provinces. In their assigned countries, chiefs of university hospital infectious disease departments spearhead "technical cooperation" efforts, and some have taken the initiative of creating their own NGOs to be more effective "actors" on the terrain. American universities, such as Harvard, University of Pennsylvania, Columbia, and others, similarly manage treatment programs for entire countries.

The shift to mass HIV treatment has raised new challenges. Proper medical management of HIV treatment requires medical record-keeping and ensuring that patients fully adhere to their treatments. Thus, as access to anti-retrovirals expands, so will the medical apparatus required to document and monitor patients' response to the drugs. Massive HIV interventions and the mass treatment programs they harbor are now faced with the large-scale bio-political challenge of classifying populations and managing their well-being in the most intimate detail. This requires mastering the logistics of deploying the technologies and commodities to do so, in places where the state does not reliably carry out biopolitical functions associated with ensuring population health.

Antiretroviral programs are likely to be the only significant interaction that many citizens in Africa—or indeed in most of the developing world—have with a complex administrative apparatus, one that parodies the modern welfare State we in the North take for granted. Three elements are visible in this apparatus: narrative and documentary practices for obtaining, record-ing, and tracking individuals' identities and experience; drugs; and forms of bodily discipline, such as adherence to drug treatment or practice of safer sex. I refer to this linkage of practices, commodities, and bodies in specific ways as "therapeutic citizenship" to underscore how it also confers on individuals specific rights (to health, in this case) as well as responsibilities (such as not infecting others).[8]

Increasingly, HIV programs have taken on the basic functions normally guaranteed by the state, albeit only for the individuals they enroll. The fram-ing of AIDS as a humanitarian crisis is empirically justified; however, doing so mobilizes a range of political and therapeutic technologies. Technologies of management, accountability, and coordination are deployed alongside antiretrovirals, food aid, school programs for orphans, and counseling to be abstinent, faithful, or use condoms. These more intimate technologies tar-get the way in which we care for our bodies, constitute our families, talk to our lovers, raise our children, and live out our sexuality. Under the rubric of AIDS, these technologies effectively constitute a kind of parallel therapeutic state. As epidemiological exception and as humanitarian emergency, through the deployment of these technologies, AIDS has enabled a form of what may be called "government-by-exception" (Nguyen 2009a). This is a republic of kinds, something that this book has called a "republic of therapy."

Exception requires that business no longer be conducted as usual and also that "exceptional" populations be constituted through interventions, which, as I have shown in this book, deploy technologies of government that keep people alive and produce new ways of life. Humanitarian interventions express a geographic logic as they group together populations to be protected or saved in refugee camps, war zones, or territories devastated by a catastrophic event. In contrast, this kind of "government-by-exception" requires the enrollment, or calling-into-being, of specific groups to be saved by foreign agents through the deployment of specific diagnostic technologies among populations of otherwise sovereign lands.

This government-by-exception is, at this point, exercised by a consortium of NGOs, foreign donor governments, Northern universities, hospitals, research institutes, churches, pharmaceuticals firms, and even the American military. It is they who now administer life-saving treatment for millions living with HIV in Africa and, indeed, in other parts of the world, through tangled organizational webs that ensure distribution of money, drugs, and resources. The tangle reflects complicated institutional arrangements that bind implementing agencies (subcontractors of development assistance, foundations, NGOs, and so on) to national governments and to foreign publics to whom they must prove that their aid money is achieving results. Through complicated organizational charts and an excessive rhetoric of "partnership" and "national capacity building," NGOs, American universities, and European hospitals channel therapeutic sovereignty. They directly govern the lives of populations with HIV and, in fact, exercise the power of life or death over them. Today, well-meaning humanitarians and development managers barely out of school shuttle in and out of Abidjan and other African cities, unaware of and largely unaccountable to the lives that are at stake. Anger at this situation has been expressed to me in terms of nostalgia for the colonial past because, at least then, one knew whom to fight and what was at stake. People gave their lives to achieve sovereignty in these postcolonial lands. Today, it seems, the only way to maintain that sovereignty would be to let themselves die.

It is too early, in this story of lives lost and lives saved, to ascertain how this curious situation will play out over time. The dream of a better future for one's children remains alive for the people I have profiled in this book and for many others, but it is one tempered by a lucid awareness that the global economic order has stacked the odds against them.

NOTES

1. The 2006 census places the city's population at slightly over five million; it is the second-largest city in West Africa after Lagos and is a major port that supplies not only Côte-d'Ivoire but land-locked Burkina Faso, Mali, and Niger to the north. Although Côte-d'Ivoire's first president Félix Houphouët-Boigny moved the political capital to his hometown of Yamoussoukro in the center of the country, the government remains concentrated in Abidjan, which is also the economic capital of the region.

2. This book adds to a large body of literature that includes several important ethnographic monographs on HIV. An early edited volume (Lindenbaum and Herdt 1992) as well as the seminal work of Farmer 1992, 2004a, 2004b, based on ethnographic fieldwork in Haiti, demonstrated the importance of cultural studies and ethnography to understanding the HIV epidemic. Other studies, such as Setel's 1999 study of AIDS in Tanzania and the sociological and historical approaches of Webb 1997 and Barnett and Whiteside 2003, explored the links between HIV's epidemiology and social and economic structure on the continent. A number of ethnographic studies of HIV in Africa have been published in the last ten years. Booth 2003 is the first full-length book study of the response to the epidemic and focuses on Kenya and the "technical difficulties" that afflicted attempts to implement international policy. Fassin's 2007 study of AIDS in South Africa examines the epidemic in the context of that country's political and economic history. Thornton 2008 provides a groundbreaking synthesis of anthropology and epidemiology that focuses on the role of sexual networks and demonstrates how these mediate the influence of culture and political economy on HIV epidemics. I have made a similar argument about Côte-d'Ivoire (Nguyen 2005).

3. Gibbal, Le Bris, Marie, Osmont, and Salem 1982 provides an early overview of urban ethnography in Africa, examining how the city is produced in everyday life and

practice. This approach, which is also that of the majority of the historians, sociologists, and anthropologists of Abidjan I cite in this book, reflects the influence of the French Marxist philosopher Henri Lefebvre and his argument (first published in French in 1947) that while we may take for granted the spaces we inhabit, they are in fact the product of social relations and forms of domination that can be decoded through an analysis of everyday life. See Lefebvre 1991, 1995 for English translations. Anglophone anthropology has been influenced by Lefebvre through the work of De Certeau 2002.

4. I am particularly indebted to the French Institute for Development Research Centre (IRD) in Petit-Bassam, and to Laurent Vidal, for graciously welcoming me and allowing me access to their documentation center.

5. Suspension of habeas corpus, extraordinary rendition, and the Guantanamo prison camp for "enemy combatants" that the United States unilaterally exempted from the Geneva Convention rules are the most notable examples. See, for instance, Aradau 2007 and Huysmans 2004.

6. Some of the ethnographic material presented in the first half of the book has been previously published: see Nguyen 2002, 2004, 2009a, and 2009b.

7. See, for example, Fink 2009 for a harrowing account of triage in a New Orleans hospital in the wake of Hurricane Katrina. A useful recent review of triage can be found in Iverson and Moskop 2007.

Notes to Chapter 1: Testimonials That Bind

1. Cordell and Piché 1992; Cordell, Gregory, and Piché 1996; Blion and Bredeloup 1997.

2. Fees for attending public primary and secondary schools were introduced in the 1980s throughout the developing world as a result of World Bank- and IMF-mandated structural readjustment programs, which advocated cost recovery through user fees.

3. See Connelly 2008 for an authoritative history of family planning.

4. Kinship is a fundamental category of anthropological analysis and was classically taken to represent the layering of social organization, understood in abstract and functional terms, over biological relatedness. See, for example, Radcliffe-Brown and Forde 1950 for an African consideration, and Fox 1967 for a magisterial overview. Since the 1970s, however, this has been replaced by approaches that have increasingly problematized the dichotomy assumed in the study of kinship between nature and culture, most recently through the example of assisted reproduction. See Peletz 1995 for an overview of the literature, Faubion 1996 for a review article that offers critical assessment, and Carsten 2003 for a recent discussion that stresses "relatedness" as a more appropriate category of analysis.

5. It has been argued that as a result of the Ivoirian "economic miracle" of the 1970s, which I describe further in chapter 6, new-found wealth led to an explosion of sexual promiscuity and prostitution, which helped establish the city as the AIDS epidemic's West African epicenter (Gould 1993). This particular explanation has not been contested, but is too simplistic and may, for example, discount the role of widespread

transfusion practices in amplifying the epidemic in the context of Abidjan's relatively westernized medical system. But the question of where "it" started and "how" it spread obscures a more basic issue: that one of the necessary preconditions for spread to occur is not migration, but the steep gradients of social inequality that drive the poor to migrate to the cities, and how those gradients structured sexual networks (see Thornton 2008 and chapter 7 of this book) and exacerbated biological vulnerabilities, notably by limiting access to diagnosis and treatment for other sexually transmitted infections, which are important cofactors of HIV transmission.

6. In 1997–98, adult HIV prevalence in Burkina Faso was estimated to be just over 7 percent; subsequently, in 2003 UNAIDS (published 2004) estimated this to be 4.2 percent, while a national household survey with HIV testing by consent found the rate to be 1.8 percent (Institut National de la Statistique, Ministère de la Lutte contre le Sida [Côte d'Ivoire], and ORC Macro 2005). The drop in the HIV rate was not unique to Burkina, as it was due to new methods used to extrapolate from surveys of specific "sentinel" groups, ranging from women receiving antenatal care to the general population. I discuss the reasons for this in the conclusion of this book.

7. Such studies involved drawing blood from select groups—such as pregnant women, those seeking treatment for sexually transmitted diseases, hospital ward patients, or even "high-risk groups" like truck drivers—and extrapolating the observed rates of HIV infection to the general population.

8. Social marketing refers to using free market methods to distribute socially useful goods—such as condoms, oral rehydration solutions for diarrhea, and so on—at a subsidized price. Resellers buy the goods cheaply, and make money by reselling them. Demand is spurred by marketing campaigns.

9. See Smith 2003 for an ethnographic discussion of per diems in Nigeria.

10. Olivier de Sardan (2005) uses the term explicitly while other analysts of African politics use similar concepts to offer a critique both of the application of the Western term "corruption" and redistributive practices organized within and around the state in Africa: notable examples are Bayart 1993 and Bayart, Stephen, and Hibou 1999. See also Olivier de Sardan 1999 on moral economies and corruption in West Africa and Smith 2001 for an anthropological examination of kinship and moral economy in the context of "corruption" in Nigeria. Elyachar 2005 is an important study focusing on NGOs and economic empowerment in Egypt that provides ethnographic and analytic perspective on moral and informal economies (see also chapter 6).

11. I explore the basis for this interpretation in chapter 7.

12. For historical accounts, Rosenberg 1992 is the classical reference for the Euro-American context; for studies that encompass epidemics in Africa, see Ranger and Slack 1995; Hays 1998; and Watts 1997. The seminal references in anthropology are Farmer's 1992 ethnography of the emergence of HIV in Haiti and Briggs and Mantini-Briggs's 2003 chronicle of a cholera epidemic in Venezuela and the subtle ways in which racism shaped perceptions of the epidemic, its "scientific" quantification, and indeed the way it evolved.

13. Initially, homosexuals, injection drug-users, blood-product recipients, and, it was erroneously believed, Haitians. The literature on stigma and the cultural dimensions of the response in the early years of the epidemic is vast and largely concerns the United States, the United Kingdom, France, and Australia; see, for instance, Bayer 1991; Crimp 1988; Patton 1990; Pollak 1988; Treichler 1987; Verghese 1995; and Watney 1994.

14. Western, modern, or scientific medicine is generally referred to by anthropologists and other social scientists as "biomedicine" to distinguish from other medical traditions (such as traditional Chinese medicine or Ayurveda) that do not ground medical knowledge and practice in biology. The concept of medicalization is used in social science to refer to the growing importance of biomedicine in various aspects of everyday life that were not previously viewed and managed as medical problems, the cardinal example being childbirth. Sociologists such as Irving Zola (1972) classically referred to medicalization as a form of social control (see also Conrad and Schneider 1980), while the anthropologist Michael Taussig (1980) argued medicalization was a form of ideology used to mask economic domination. Since these early studies, anthropologists and sociologists have drawn on the French philosopher Michel Foucault to argue for a more nuanced approach that takes into account both domination and resistance to biomedicine in a range of settings (Lock and Gordon 1988; Lindenbaum and Lock 1993). See Rose 2007 for a useful and succinct review.

15. The third revision of the American Psychiatric Association's "Diagnostics and Statistics Manual" removed homosexuality as a disease in 1980. See Bayer 1987 for an account.

16. See Seidel 1993 and Gruskin, Tomasevski, and Hendriks 1996 for an introduction to GIPA. A more recent study of GIPA, through an ethnographic account of its effects on South African AIDS activism, is Robins 2006.

17. The text of the letter was published in the local newspaper *L'Observateur Paalga*; the translation is mine from the text copied into my field notes.

18. I discuss this further in chapter 7.

19. I discuss this further in chapter 6.

20. Matthieu resurfaced three years later, in 1999, embroiled in the assassination of the leading opposition journalist Norbert Zongo in 1998. Matthieu claimed the Burkinabè government hired him to carry out the assassination, but then he recanted at the last moment, stating that opposition forces had paid him to frame the president's régime.

Notes to Chapter 2: Confessional Technologies

1. I elaborate on this clinical experiment in chapter 4.

2. Foucault is translated and quoted by Taylor 2009, 30, in an excellent overview of confession in Foucault. The original references are Foucault 1978, especially chap. 1, and Foucault 1997a, 1997b.

3. See Pigg 2001 for an anthropological analysis of HIV prevention in Nepal and Pigg

2005 for an important critical assessment of how these workshops disseminated "new facts of life."

4. Anthropologists have stressed how this reflects how development assistance is framed in ways that make it difficult to contest, drawing on Foucault's theories of discourse and micropolitics to argue that this marks an insidious political strategy; see Escobar 1995 and Ferguson 1994 for important monographs, and Fisher 1997 for a review. Cheater 1999 offers a comprehensive anthropological examination of "empowerment," Riles 2001 provides an important ethnography of the material practice of this new form of transnational politics, and Li 2007 is an important new study from Indonesia; for an "insider account," see Eyben 2000.

5. Harvey 2005 offers a succinct and informative account of the rise of neoliberalism. See Cruikshank 1999 for an important study of empowerment in the context of welfare reform in the United States. The "new development" is discussed in Gardner and Lewis 1995, 103–38; see also Cooper and Packard 1997. Post-Fordism is comprehensively discussed in Harvey 1994 and A. Amin 1994; see E. Martin 1995 for an anthropological study of post-Fordism in American culture.

6. Stirrat (2000) provides an ethnographic analysis of the rationalizing and modernizing "cultures of consultancy" in international development and links these to older colonial and missionary projects, while O'Malley, Nguyen, and Lee (1996) describe the role of NGOs in the AIDS response.

7. This was not surprising, given the profound effect of the French tainted-blood scandal of the mid-1980s on the perception of the medical establishment and the state in France. The scandal led to the imprisonment of senior physicians of the National Blood Bank, as well as the indictment of the minister of health and the prime minister at the time. The scandal was cleverly exploited by the far-right National Front party to inaccurately link tainted blood with immigration (Kramer 1993). One of Juan's field officers, a British man, referred to the money France was spending on AIDS in Africa as "guilt money" for the tainted-blood scandal.

8. Michèle Martin (2003) shows this in a fascinating study that examines the introduction of female telephone operators by Bell Canada in the early twentieth century.

9. As we shall see, "international best practice" and the urgency with which interventions were reproduced meant that many practices were disseminated before their longer-term effects on communities could become clear.

10. See Rogers 1970, but also Lee 2002.

11. A recent special issue of the *Journal of Religion in Africa* has a number of contributions that explore the intersection of religion and AIDS, but they do not deal specifically with confession: for an overview see Becker and Geissler 2007. See also Robins 2006.

Notes to Chapter 3: Soldiers of God

1. Having served on British ships since the eighteenth century, some coastal tribes in present-day Liberia and Western Côte-d'Ivoire are known as Krou or Kroumen.

2. David Shank (1994, 91–96) makes the case for Harris's involvement in a coup attempt alongside Edward Blyden, the African American colonist sympathetic to the "natives," who was one of the fathers of pan-Africanism. See also Shank 1999.

3. The historical ethnography of this "prophetic" belt constitutes an important strand of French anthropology. The early work of Marc Augé, initially influenced by the Marxist anthropology of the "modes of production" school (see Foster-Carter 1978; Godelier 1975, 1978; Asad and Wolpe 1976; Asad 1985; Geschiere and Raatgever 1985; Raatgever 1985), analyzed the kinship structure of the ethnic groups that lived along the coast and lagoons, the so-called "lagunar tribes." This school viewed kinship as a form of "ideology," that is, as the representation a society makes of itself and the theory of power this expresses (Augé 1974, 1975). Gruénais (1984) draws critically on Augé for his study of the Mossi in Burkina Faso. While Augé is usually credited in French for the concept of "therapeutic itineraries" as a method for ethnographically tracking sufferers' patterns of resort (Augé and Herzlich 1983; see also Janzen 1982), he is better known for his more literary ethnographies of Parisian urban memory and the "non-spaces" of hypermodernity (for instance, see Augé 1992, 1997). Nonetheless his continued ethnographic engagement with Côte-d'Ivoire drew him to contemporary prophets (Augé and Colleyn 1995), following groundbreaking earlier studies by Rouch 1963 and Piault 1975. This work was continued by his student Jean-Pierre Dozon (1995), on which this account draws extensively. For a dissenting view that sees the legacy of Harris and prophetic cults less favorably, see Perrot 1996.

4. The "black yam movement" involved the destruction of yams favored by colonial traders, resulting in starvation in parts of the colony.

5. Another example is the Congolese Zionist Kimbangu Kitawala.

6. For discussions of prophecy, anticipation, and the culture of Ivoirian politics, see Augé 1994 and Mary 1997. See Bureau 1996 for a full study of the Harrist church. The following historical and ethnographic studies of religious movements in Francophone West Africa also provide valuable context: Laurent 1998; Mary 1999; Paulme 1963; and Sirven 1967. Da Silva 1993 offers an anthropological overview of African Independent Churches, while Ranger 1986's seminal review of religious movements and politics in sub-Saharan Africa contextualizes Ivoirian history within a broader African dynamic.

7. For instance, in Côte-d'Ivoire, where they are called *tontines*, these thrift associations are common and are most often made up of women who sell in markets.

8. Key references in this debate are Balandier 1985; Banton 1965, 1973; Epstein 1961, 1967; Gluckman 1940; Little 1962; Parkin 1966; and Schwab 1970.

9. With the notable exception of Balandier 1985.

10. See Jézéquel 1999 on African theatre in colonial French West Africa; P. Martin (1985) addresses issues of colonial sociality through leisure activities in colonial French Equatorial Africa's capital of Brazzaville. Hunt (1994) raises issues of colonial mobility, letter writing, and self-fashioning in the Belgian Congo—issues that are further developed in Hunt 1999.

11. Conklin (1997, 1998) provides important historical insight on the links between the French "civilizing" mission, voluntary association, and domesticity in French Africa. See also Berron 1980 for an excellent early study that is critical of the opposition between "tradition" and "modernity" in Côte-d'Ivoire. Mamdani (for example, 2001) makes a similar and influential argument in his extensive writings against colonial determinist views of political consciousness in Africa, although he refers largely to the British colonial experience.

12. Anthropologists have written a number of studies on the subject of religion and AIDS in Africa (Garner 2000; Smith 2004; Pfeiffer 2002, 2004; Becker and Geissler 2007) and have stressed how religion mediates representations and practices of the disease in terms of local political and economic context, sometimes at cross-purposes with what international agencies intend in their AIDS awareness efforts. In the public health and medical literature, there has been an explosion of interest in the topic since 2000, stemming from the awareness that religious communities play an important part in caring for the ill and affected and from the strong interest of U.S. President George W. Bush's administration (2000–2008) in involving "faith-based organizations" in AIDS work.

13. I will return to the reasons for this in chapters 5 and 6.

14. Prince (2007) and Kalofonos (2008) have reported similar phenomena.

15. I will discuss this issue in the following chapter.

16. A telling inversion of AIDS marches in Northern countries, where marchers seek out their own sponsors and the proceeds go to the organization.

17. This is described in a journalistic profile of Joséphine Oupoh, with whom I worked at the Abidjan clinic (Pompey 1999, 18). The relationship between kinship and power, initially posed by Morgan (1877) was a major concern of colonial anthropology, particularly in light of the British policy of indirect rule through "tribal headmen" and its lesser-known French counterpart (Crowder 1964). It is in this political context that the "tribes without rulers" emerged as an anthropological problem (Fortes 2008; Middleton and Tait 1958) and a source of theorizing about the origin of the state (see Clastres 1982).

18. I use the term in the manner Dorward (1974) used it to describe how in colonial Nigeria, despite British perceptions of Nigerians being shaped by stereotypes of "tribes" and imagined cultural attributes, a working misunderstanding nonetheless ensued as Nigerians adapted to colonial rule. A similar process occurred in colonial Côte-d'Ivoire and will be further explored in chapter 5.

Notes to Chapter 4: Life Itself

1. The sociologist Nikolas Rose (2006, 3) defines the "politics of life itself," in an influential book of the same name, as a form of politics "concerned with our growing capacities to control, manage, engineer, reshape, and modulate the very capacity of human beings as living creatures." I use the term somewhat differently, to examine what came to be at stake with the promise of treatment.

2. A full-length study of this can be found in Steve Epstein's sociological study of how AIDS activists in America helped shaped the emerging clinical science of HIV (S. Epstein 1996); see also Brown 1997 for an account of American AIDS activism as an exemplar of radical democratic practice. Biomedical forms of citizenship have been described by medical anthropologists and sociologists in other settings. Adriana Petryna, for instance, introduced the term "biological citizenship" in her ethnographic study of the aftermath of the Chernobyl nuclear disaster to highlight how its victims mobilized evidence of their damaged biology to make compensation claims (Petryna 2002). Rose and Novas also use the term in a more general sense to refer to how "citizenship projects organized in the name of 'health'" (Rose 2006, 24) are increasingly articulated in biomedical terms (Rose and Novas 2004). Heath, Rapp, and Taussig (2004) have used the term "genetic citizenship" in a similar manner.

3. The seminal historical account of the Tuskegee experiments can be read in Jones 1993. Washington (2006) contextualizes Tuskegee within a long history of medical experimentation on African Americans. Wendland (2008) provides a detailed review of the controversy over the Ugandan PMTCT trials and draws on her own work in Africa to provide an important critique of the issues.

4. See Institute of Medicine, Board on Population Health and Public Health Practice 2005.

5. Petryna (2005), in her study of globalizing clinical trials in Eastern Europe, speaks of "ethical variability" in reference to a similar phenomenon; a fuller study has just been published (Petryna 2009).

6. A normal T4 cell count is over six hundred; with less than fifty cells, patients are at high risk of serious opportunistic infections and death within the year.

7. The first generation of protease inhibitors have a short half-life in the body and required an almost military discipline to ensure they were effective; this is no longer the case with newer treatment regimens that use pharmacologic "boosting" strategies to ensure a longer half-life, doing away with the need to adhere to strict schedules.

8. Fassin (2001) describes what can be called a "biologization" of France's political asylum policies, which made it increasingly difficult to obtain asylum on political grounds, even as "humanitarian exceptions" were made for those with illnesses such as HIV, what Ticktin (2006) has called the "violence of humanitarianism." Both point to the political dimensions of these humanitarian exceptions, drawing on the work of Agamben (1995, 2005) and the German political philosopher Carl Schmitt.

9. Because triple therapy completely suppresses HIV's replication, it allows the immune system to recover over time. Intermittent triple therapy, that is, taking three drugs for a year and then stopping, could be expected to "buy time" for the patient with a minimal risk of acquiring resistance to the drugs. In contrast, double therapy does not completely suppress the virus, allowing it to become resistant, and with only fleeting benefit for the patient's immune system; essentially, after six months, the

drugs would be useless. At the time I was in Abidjan, the notion that intermittent triple therapy could be a treatment strategy was not discussed, although I was aware of it from my practice in Montreal, where patients regularly requested to go on "drug holidays." In the next few years, the "on and off" strategy—referred to as "structured treatment interruptions"—gained support and was tested in a number of important international clinical trials that proved that it was inferior to continuous triple therapy but still better than treatment with two drugs. These are reviewed in Eron 2008, S267–68.

10. Using only two drugs allows HIV to continue replicating and develop resistance to the drugs, as mentioned above. Even worse, once the virus becomes resistant to one drug, it is often resistant to other drugs in the same class—a phenomenon known as "cross-resistance"—that makes them of no use in a new cocktail. This led to a paradoxical historical injustice for patients who were treated with only two drugs in the early 1990s (as was the case in North America and Europe) and found themselves saddled with a resistant virus and little or no treatment options within a few years, while those who were treated a bit later, from 1995, often got three drugs and were therefore much better off over the long term. By 2008, however, the advent of new antiretroviral drug classes and new drugs in the older classes had leveled the playing field somewhat for those who had had inadequate treatment early on, when three drugs were not yet available. However these new drugs are not yet available in developing countries because of their expense.

11. This account can be contrasted to that of medical anthropologist Joao Biehl (2007), who describes a parallel evolution of the "ideal form of communitarian sociality" (63) embodied by HIV groups in Brazil, pointing to how a "micropolitics of patienthood" enacts a "performance" of citizenship (120–24). Triage in Brazil was also a reality, despite a model national treatment program. Biehl observed the "coexistence in the triage room of dying patients with recovering patients, who had to assume the role of caretakers" (276) and followed patients who, with the treatments, resumed life. Although "physically well," these patients were "economically dead" (353). Biehl describes the types of biomedical citizenship in the era of AIDS therapies as "processes of individual and group becoming . . . taking place through medicines and multiple sites, relations and intensities—fields of immanence. It is within this circuitry, as it unequally determines life chances, that AIDS survivors articulate their 'plastic power' (instead of a given truth or life form) and invent a domesticity and health to live in and by" (361).

Notes to Chapter 5: Biopower

1. I elaborate on the impact of this "deschooling" in chapter 6.
2. It was during these years that yellow fever was being eradicated in Havana and Rio by attacking the *aedes aegyptii* mosquito vector (Cooper and Kiple 1993).
3. It is likely that, living in an endemic zone, Africans would not have been as susceptible because of acquired immunity. The historical literature on yellow fever in the

Americas suggests that epidemics broke out either with the influx of large numbers of susceptible individuals or when the pathogen was imported to areas that had previously not been exposed to the disease (see Cooper and Kiple 1993).

4. Wondji (1972) queries whether this rhetoric corresponded to actual panic among the settlers, citing informants who recalled the Europeans' relative calm, noting that a "funereal rhetoric" was à propos for the settlers for whom colonial service was imbued with a sense of mission. Dramatic missives of disease, he argues, served to deepen the "apostolic conscience" of settlers. While the point is well taken, the toll the epidemics took suggests that these reports can not be dismissed as a colonial hysteria.

5. See also Curtin 1992 and, for a succinct overview, Hannaway 1993. Le Pape (1985) explains the impact on Abidjan. See also Frenkel and Western 1988 for an example from Sierra Leone.

6. From the report of the municipal commission examining the project of relocating the indigenous quarter of Old Cocody, quoted in Le Pape 1985, 303; translation mine.

7. The historian and sociologist of science Bruno Latour has written an important critical study of the "pasteurization" of France (Latour 1988; for an earlier version, see Latour 1986). Studies of the colonial reception of Pasteur's ideas, some of which are cited further below, are Bado 1996; Dozon 1985b, 1987, 1991; Marcovich 1988; and Moulin 1992, 1996.

8. The success of Jamin's 1926 campaign to contain an epidemic of sleeping sickness in Togo, conducted with military discipline and systematicity, played a large part in winning over colonial administrators to Pasteurian ideas (Dozon 1985b).

9. As recounted in Domergues-Cloarec 1986 and Dozon 1985b.

10. Tirefort (1983, 1992, and 1999) contextualizes this ethnographic urge through accounts of colonial life for French settlers in Côte-d'Ivoire.

11. In addition to Chauveau and Dozon 1987, studies of French colonial ethnography are Bender 1965; Dory 1984, 1992; Dozon 1985a; Sibeaud 1994; and Wooten 1993.

12. This argument is made in great detail in Chauveau and Dozon 1985a, drawing on material published by the same authors in 1985. Reference to the self-justifying labeling of "natives" and the particularly apt term "working misunderstanding" is once again drawn from Dorward's 1974 discussion of a similar process in relations between the British and the Tiv of Northwestern Nigeria.

13. For a full account, see Chauveau 1987. Weiskel 1980 gives the most detailed precolonial history of the Baoulé, but takes the ethnicity at face value. A similar argument for the colonial constitution of an Ivoirian ethnic group is Dozon 1985a.

14. See Challenor 1979 and Derrick 1983 for historical examinations of the "colonial clerk."

15. Other ethnographic studies of Baoulé kinship and demography are Étienne and Étienne 1968; M. Étienne 1979; Mary 1974; and Perrot 1987. For accounts of the emergence of an "indigenous" planter class, see Fauré and Médard 1982; Fréchou 1955; Hecht 1984; Gastellu and Yapi 1982; and Groff 1987.

16. While this discussion focuses on the specific issue of housing, it is informed by work that has shown the historical importance of urbanization in Africa more generally; see Coquery-Vidrovitch 1991; Cooper 1983, 1994. In addition to the references cited in the text, I acknowledge the work of Bernus 1962; Chaléard and Dubresson 1989; Diabaté, n.d.; Dureau 1985; Haeringer 1969a, 1969b; Kipré 1988; Manou-Savina 1989; Yapi-Diahou 1994; and Zan 1976.

17. The following section draws mainly on Le Pape 1997; see also Fetter 1987 for a more general discussion of African census data.

18. The high-modernist plans the postcolonial government had for Abidjan, including a new street grid, triumphal avenues, and a monorail, were lavishly laid out in 1969 in a fascinating special issue of *Urbanisme français*; see Depret and Cames 1969.

19. Growth would actually accelerate during the boom of the 1960s and 1970s. Despite a subsequent slowdown with the crisis of the 1990s, in 2000 the city's population was estimated at between 4 and 6.6 million; either way, a far cry from the 3 million predicted at the time of the *Plans d'urbanisme*. See Roland et al. 1969, 26. This did not emerge as a "planning" problem then—likely because colonial authorities never conceived of the growing urban masses as anything other than cheap labor that had to be disciplined temporarily through the ordinances described in the next chapter.

20. Armand 1988, 265; see also Dubresson and Yapi-Diahou 1988.

21. For an account, see Cazemajor 1981.

22. Le Pape, Vidal, and Yapi-Diahou 1991, 10–11.

23. See Antoine, Dubresson, and Manou-Savina 1987 for an ethnographic account of Abidjan housing, and Antoine (1988), who describes housing strategies in more detail.

24. Hacking (1986, 223) initially discusses this in light of a historical and philosophical examination of the introduction of new ways in which the nineteenth-century state sought to map its population: "Even national and provincial censuses amazingly show that the categories into which people fall change every ten years. Social change creates new categories of people, but the counting is no mere report of developments. It elaborately, often philanthropically, creates new ways for people to be," and, as he notes, "people come spontaneously to fit their categories." He elaborates this argument further in a thoughtful discussion of the molding of child abuse. Hacking 1999, 125–63.

Notes to Chapter 6: The Crisis

1. See M. Cohen 1973, 1974; and Zolberg 1964.

2. I borrow the term "promissory notes" from Wittrock's discussion of modernity in Wittrock 2000.

3. Studies of the Ivoirian crisis include de Miras 1980; Joshi, Lubell, and Mouly 1976; Vimard and N'Cho 1995; and Vidal 1990.

4. The most notable critic of structural adjustment is the Nobel Prize economist and former World Bank vice president and chief economist, Joseph Stiglitz (2003); a par-

ticularly devastating insider account is Perkins 2005. See also Chossudovsky 1997 and Davis 2007.

5. The effect of the crisis and the structural adjustment that followed it are documented in Aka 1991; Akindès 1991; Duranson 1994; Grootaert and Kanbur 1995; Grootaert, Kanbur, and Oh 1997; Jarret and Mahieu 1991; Kadet 1999; and Kanbur 1990.

6. It is worth underscoring here that the number of dependents is proportional to income rather than actual kin relations.

7. Vidal 1990; Le Pape, Vidal, and Yapi-Diahou 1991; Vidal 1997.

8. Interestingly, destruction of informal neighborhoods began again after 1995 once the economy improved, with the destruction of the shantytown of "Washington."

9. Studies of schooling in Côte-d'Ivoire are Clignet and Foster 1966; Clignet 1966, 1967; Désalmand 1986; Gardiner 1985; Gibbal 1974a; and Le Pape and Vidal 1987.

10. Le Pape 1986; Ginoux-Pouyaud 1996.

11. This shows the historical context of the phenomenon of trading favors for sex, which has become a major preoccupation in the context of the HIV epidemic, where it is seen to be a major force driving the epidemic among young girls. See, for example, Silberschmidt and Rasch 2001; Luke 2003; Leclerc-Madlala 2003; Laga, Schwartlander, Pisani, Sow, and Carael 2001; Maganja, Maman, Groves, and Mbwambo 2007; Hawkin, Price, and Mussa 2009; and Hunter 2002, 2006.

12. The initial conception of "informal" referred to economic exchange that occurred "outside" the formal institutions that in modern societies regulate economic activity, most notably the state but also the financial sector (see, for instance, Hart 1973; International Labour Office 1972). This has been challenged in contexts where the relationship between the state and "society" has not crystallized in the same manner as in Western societies. In most African countries, the informal economy is larger than the formal economy. Roitman (1990) engages a critique of both liberal and Marxist views of informal economy, drawing on Africa as an example (see also Hansen 2004 for a consideration of the informal economy in Lusaka; Bazenguissa-Ganga and MacGaffey 2000 for a monograph examining transnational trade between Central Africa and Europe; and Roitman 2004 for a book-length study focusing on Cameroun). The account that follows is in line with the arguments of Roitman (2004, 19) in recognizing that in Abidjan the parallel economy has come to be "at the heart of productive economic life" and is corroborated by Newell's examination of the "moral economy of theft" in Abidjan (Newell 2006). A moral economy, as discussed in chapter 1, characterizes aspects of parallel economies; however, as Roitman 1990 points out, the distinction between the two makes assumptions (for instance about what is "moral") which may be difficult to sustain. Unlike Roitman and others, in this account, I focus on the forms of selfhood that emerge in the parallel economy rather than on specifically economic, social, or political aspects and use the term "moral economy" as explored in chapter 1 as a lens for viewing conflicting perceptions of debt, reciprocity, and social ties in specific contexts.

13. See Mbembe 2002 for a discussion of "African modes of self-writing," which draws on this concept.

14. Zouglou dance involves a series of motions where the dancer's body language asks "why?," pleading to the right, then to the left, and finally upward because only God knows the answer (Bahi 1997); see also Gnahoré 1992.

15. English-speaking Africanists may be more familiar with the term *matatu*, which is used in Nairobi.

16. For the poor, prohibitive fees for opening accounts make regular banking inaccessible. Caisses populaires (or peoples' banks) were introduced in West Africa by the Québec Fédération des Caisses populaires Desjardins. Like the Grameen Banks in Bangladesh, these banks for the poor have spread throughout West Africa and have made "microcredit" a reality in many poor communities.

17. The current president of the Second Republic, historian Laurent Gbagbo, was for many years the lone opposition figure to Houphouët and is himself Bété.

18. *Envoyé special*, France-2 Télévision, rebroadcast on TV5 on 28 March 2001.

19. See Kouakou N'Guessan 1983; Le Pape and Vidal 1982; Manou-Savina and Dubresson 1985.

20. See, for instance, Barnett and Whiteside 2003; O'Manique 2004; Poku and Whiteside 2002.

Notes to Chapter 7: Uses and Pleasures

1. For background on the city's demographic history, see Antoine and Herry 1981; Antoine 1988; and Antoine, Dubresson, and Manou-Savina 1987.

2. See Rouch and Bernus 1957 for a study of prostitution in colonial Abidjan.

3. For a consideration of how the devaluation signaled a change in Franco-African relations, see G. Martin 1995. Crook 1997 discusses the impact of devaluation on Ivoirian politics, and Mahieu 1995 contextualizes the impact of the devaluation in light of previous structural adjustment policies.

4. The subject of homosexuality in Africa has recently been the object of two book-length studies: see Epprecht 2008 and Hoad 2007. While there are currently no ethnographies of homosexuality in Africa, Boellstorff 2005 provides a full-length study of sexuality, nationhood, and gay and lesbian identity in Indonesia. The notion of "dubbing" (as in dubbing foreign-language films) an identity by drawing on foreign sources offers an alternative perspective on the material I will discuss below; however, most of my informants did not link sexuality to identity.

5. The acronym of the French high-speed train: Train à Grande Vitesse.

6. See Daddieh 2001 for an analysis that frames Ivoirité and civil strife in terms of the "unfinished business" of Houphouët's succession. See also the articles published in a special issue of *Politique africaine* in 2000 dedicated to ethnonationalism in Côte-d'Ivoire (Akindès 2000; Campbell 2000; Chauveau 2000; Dozon 2000; and Losch 2000). The issue includes an article by the Franco-Canadian journalist Guy-André

Kieffer (2000), who was abducted four years later and is believed to have been assassinated (Reporters without Borders 2009). Le Pape and Vidal 2002 brings together accounts of the "terrible year" leading up to and following the coup.

7. See Bassett 2004; Hellweg 2004, 2009.

8. See Posel 2008 for a compelling account of sex, confession, and citizenship in the New South Africa.

Notes to Conclusion

1. A more general statement of this argument can be found in Comaroff (2007) who links the "biopolitics of AIDS" to the global neoliberal order. In contrast, Abélès (2006) argues that the practices of triage I describe here are a "politics of survival" that has emerged with the breakdown of the liberal project of the modern state.

2. In the context of international interventions, McFalls (2007, 1–2) defines iatrogenic violence as "social disruption and political violence that results from outside intervention (military and/or 'humanitarian') intended to stop or to prevent such violence" that, he argues, "is inherent to the *formal* structure of international intervention, regardless of the substantive means, motives, or context of intervention."

3. PEPFAR, for instance, has already committed 18.5 billion U.S. dollars over the next five years, most of it on treatment, and shortly before leaving office, President George W. Bush asked to increase this to 30 billion dollars. The Global Fund has already committed 11.4 billion U.S. dollars and, according to its executive director, is aiming to triple funding for HIV to between 6 and 8 billion U.S. dollars annually by 2010 to combat HIV, tuberculosis, and malaria, much of the funds devoted to "ramping up" treatment programs. These efforts represent an unprecedented intervention on entire populations by nongovernmental organizations and foreign powers. See Coriat 2008 and Foller and Thorn 2008 for empirical analyses of the politics and political economy of the AIDS industry in the developing world.

4. The figures are from PEPFAR 2009, 44, and appear to be accurate based on conversations with Ivoirian and French officials up to June 2009. The effects of Côte-d'Ivoire's treatment program in terms of health and cost has been assessed recently in Losina, Yazdanpanah, Deuffic-Burban, Wang, Wolf, Messou, Gabillard, Seyler, Freedberg, and Anglaret 2007; and Goldie, Yazdanpanah, Losina, Weinstein, Anglaret, Walensky, and Hsu 2006.

5. Incidentally, this change determined that previous seroprevalence estimates were too high. Walker, Grassly, Garnett, Stanecki, and Ghys 2004.

6. Researchers have highlighted how resource flows targeting AIDS relief in Africa do not necessarily go directly to preventing HIV or caring for the ill and indeed how some or much of it is tied to promoting donor nations' and international organizations' political agendas around trade, intellectual property, and so forth. O'Manique 2004; Poku and Whiteside 2002; Scott 2000; Sparke 2009. More significantly, the money flowing *into* developing countries for AIDS, at least in the African context, is dwarfed by the money flowing *out* for debt servicing. This has led for calls to for-

give debt for developing countries so that the money freed up could be devoted to addressing health issues such as HIV (Kaddar and Furrer 2008); some progress on this issue has occurred (Cassimon and Van Campenhout 2007). There are reports that some countries are following the example set by mass treatment programs by dedicating portions of these new funds to providing ARVs (Shacinda 2005), demonstrating how this issue of treatment for HIV both liberates and captures capital flows.

7. Personal communication, 27 March 2009.

8. Ong (2006) argues that this form of "graduated" or differentiated citizenship is a defining feature of global neoliberalism, drawing on her fieldwork in Southeast Asia. In contrast, in this book I have argued that these differentiated citizenships are built on earlier foundations established by colonial and postcolonial dividing practices.

REFERENCES

Abélès, Marc. 2006. *Politique de la survie*. Paris: Flammarion.

Adjé, Christiane, Rachanee Cheingsong, Thierry H. Roels, Chantal Maurice, Gaston Djomand, Werner Verbiest, Kurt Hertogs et al. 2001. "High Prevalence of Genotypic and Phenotypic HIV-1 Drug-Resistant Strains among Patients Receiving Antiretroviral Therapy in Abidjan, Côte d'Ivoire." UNAIDS HIV Drug Access Initiative, Abidjan, Côte d'Ivoire. *J Acquir Immune Defic Syndr* 26, no. 5, 501–6.

Affoum, Édith Marie-Laurence. 1982. "La France et les établissements français de Côte d'Ivoire: Grand-Bassam, Assinie, Dabou (1838–1870)." Master's thesis, Faculté des lettres, arts et sciences humaines, Université nationale de Côte-d'Ivoire, Abidjan.

Agamben, Giorgio. 1995. *Homo Sacer*. Chicago: University of Chicago Press.

———. 2005. *State of Exception*. Chicago: University of Chicago Press.

Aka, Kouamé. 1991. "Restructuration du marché du travail en Côte-d'Ivoire." *Canadian Journal of African Studies* 25, no. 3, 396–416.

Akindès, Francis. 1991. "Restauration populaire et sécurité alimentaire à Abidjan." *Cahiers des sciences humaines* 27, nos. 1–2, 169–82.

———. 2000. "Inégalités sociales et régulation politique en Côte-d'Ivoire." *Politique africaine* 78, 126–41.

Amin, Ash. 1994. *Post-Fordism: A Reader*. London: Basil Blackwell.

Amin, Samir. 1967. *Le Développement du capitalisme en Cote d'Ivoire*. Paris: Les Editions de Minuit.

Amoore, Louise. 2006. "Biometric Border: Governing Mobilities in the War on Terror." *Political Geography* 25, 336–51.

Anderson, Robert T. 1971. "Voluntary Associations in History." *American Anthropologist* 73, no. 1, 209–22.

Anonymous. 1969. "Abidjan, Côte-d'Ivoire: Plans d'urbanisme." *Urbanisme Revue française* 111–12, 20–36.

Antoine, Philippe. 1988. "Comportements démographiques et urbanisation à Abidjan." *Espace populations sociétés* 2, 227–43.

Antoine, Philippe, Alain Dubresson, and Annie Manou-Savina. 1987. *Abidjan "côté cours."* Paris: Karthala.

Antoine, Philippe, and Claude Herry. 1981. *Implications du déséquilibre de la structure par âge et par sexe: Le cas d'une métropole africaine: Abidjan.* Abidjan: Centre ORSTOM de Sciences humaines.

Aradau, Claudia. 2007. "Law Transformed: Guantanamo and the 'Other' Exception." *Third World Quarterly* 28, no. 3, 489–501.

Ardener, Shirley. 1964. "The Comparative Study of Rotating Credit Associations." *Journal of the Royal Anthropological Institute* 94, 201–29.

Armand, Myriam. 1988. "Tissu urbain, tissu social: Stratégie antagonistes d'occupation de l'espace à Abidjan." *Espace populations sociétés* 2, 261–74.

Arnold, David, ed. 1996. *Warm Climates and Western Medicine: The Emergence of Tropical Medicine 1500–1900.* Amsterdam: Rodopi.

Asad, Talal. 1985. "Primitive States and the Reproduction of Production Relations: Some Problems in Marxist Anthropology." *Critique of Anthropology* 5, no. 2, 21–33.

Asad, Talal, and Harold Wolpe. 1976. "Concepts of Modes of Production." *Economy and Society* 5, no. 4, 470–506.

Atger, Paul. 1962. *La France en Côte-d'Ivoire de 1843 à 1893: Cinquante ans d'hésitations politiques et commerciales.* Dakar: Publication de la section d'Histoire de l'Université de Dakar.

Augé, Marc, ed. 1974. *La Construction du monde: Religion, représentations, idéologie.* Paris: Maspero.

———. 1975. *Théorie des pouvoirs et idéologie: Étude de cas en Côte d'Ivoire.* Paris: Hermann.

———. 1992. *Non-lieux: Introduction à une anthropologie de la surmodernité.* Paris: Éditions du Seuil.

———. 1994. "Prophetic Anticipation (Some Remarks on the Prophet-Healers of Ivory Coast)." *Journal of Social Studies* 66, 10–20.

———. 1997. *La guerre des rêves: Exercices d'ethno fiction.* Paris: Éditions du Seuil.

Augé, Marc, and Jean-Paul Colleyn. 1995. *Nkpiti: La rancune et le prophète.* Paris: Éditions de l'École des Hautes Études en Sciences Sociales.

Augé, Marc, and Claudine Herzlich. 1983. *Le Sens du mal: Anthropologie, histoire, sociologie de la maladie.* Paris: Éditions des Archives contemporaines.

Austen, Ralph A. 1993. "The Moral Economy of Witchcraft: An Essay in Comparative History." *Modernity and Its Malcontents: Ritual and Power in Postcolonial Africa*, Jean Comaroff and John Comaroff, eds., 89–110. Chicago: University of Chicago Press.

Bado, Jean-Paul. 1996. *Médecine coloniale et grandes endémies en Afrique.* Paris: Karthala.

Bahi, Boniface. 1997. "Danse et espace idéologique des jeunes de la marge." *Sociétés Africaines et diasporas* 3, 105–17.

Balandier, Georges. 1985. *Sociologie des Brazzavilles noires*, 2nd edn. Paris: Presses de la fondation nationale des sciences politiques.

Banton, Michael. 1965. "Social Alignment and Identity in a West African City." *Urbani-*

zation and Migration in West Africa, ed. Hilda Kuper, 131–47. Westport, Conn.: Greenwood Press.

———. 1973. "Urbanization and Role Analysis." *Urban Anthropology: Cross-cultural Studies of Urbanization*, ed. Aidan Southall, 43–70. New York: Oxford University Press.

Barnett, Tony, and Alan Whiteside. 2003. AIDS *in the Twenty-first Century: Disease and Globalization*. Basingstoke: Palgrave.

Bassett, Thomas J. 2004. "Containing the Donzow." *Africa Today* 50, no. 4, 31–49.

Bayart, Jean-François. 1993. *The State in Africa: The Politics of the Belly*. London: Longman Group.

Bayart, Jean-François, Ellis Stephen, and Béatrice Hibou. 1999. *The Criminalization of the State in Africa*. Indianapolis: Indiana University Press.

Bayer, Ronald. 1987. *Homosexuality and American Psychiatry*. Princeton: Princeton University Press.

———. 1991. *Private Acts, Social Consequences:* AIDS *and the Politics of Public Health*. New Brunswick, N.J.: Rutgers University Press.

Bazenguissa-Ganga, Janet, and Remy MacGaffey. 2000. *Congo-Paris: Transnational Traders on the Margins of the Law*. Bloomington: Indiana University Press.

Becker, Felicitas, and P. Wenzel Geissler. 2007. "Searching for Pathways in a Landscape of Death: Religion and AIDS in East Africa." *Journal of Religion in Africa* 37, no. 1, 1–15.

Bender, Donald. 1965. "The Development of French Anthropology." *Journal of the History of the Behavioral Sciences* 1, no. 2, 139–51.

Bernus, Edmond. 1962. "Abidjan: Note sur l'agglomération." *Bulletin de l'institut français d'Afrique noire* 24, nos. 1–2, 54–85.

Berron, Henri. 1980. *Tradition et modernisme en pays lagunaires de basse Côte-d'Ivoire*. Paris: Éditions Ophyrys.

Biehl, Joao. 2007. *Will to Live:* AIDS *Therapies and the Politics of Survival*. Princeton: Princeton University Press.

Biggs, Michael. 1999. "Putting the State on the Map: Cartography, Territory, and European State Formation." *Comparative Studies in Society and History* 41, no. 2, 374–505.

Blion, Reynald, and Sylvie Brédéloup. 1997. "La Côte-d'Ivoire dans les stratégies migratoires des Burkinabè et des Sénégalais." *Le modèle ivoirien en questions: Crises, ajustements, recompositions*, Bernard Contamin and Harris Memel-Fotê, eds., 707–38. Paris: Karthala and ORSTOM.

Boellstorff, Tom. 2005. *The Gay Archipelago: Sexuality and Nation in Indonesia*. Princeton: Princeton University Press.

Booth, Karen M. 2003. *Local Women, Global Science: Fighting* AIDS *in Kenya*. Bloomington: Indiana University Press.

Briggs, Charles L., and Clara Mantini-Briggs. 2003. *Stories in the Time of Cholera: Racial Profiling during a Medical Nightmare*. Berkeley: University of California Press.

Brown, Michael P. 1997. *Replacing Citizenship:* AIDS *Activism and Radical Democracy*. New York: Guilford Press.

Bureau, René. 1996. *Le prophète de la lagune: Les harristes de Côte-d'Ivoire*. Paris: Karthala.

Campbell, Bonnie. 1997. "Le modèle ivoirien de développement à l'épreuve de la crise." *Le modèle ivoirien en questions: Crises, ajustements, recompositions*, Bernard Contamin and Harris Memel-Fotê, eds., 37–60. Paris: Karthala and ORSTOM.

———. 2000. "Réinvention du politique en Côte-d'Ivoire." *Politique africaine* 78, 142–56.

Carsten, Janet. 2003. *After Kinship*. New York: Cambridge University Press.

Cassimon, Danny, and Bjorn Van Campenhout. 2007. "Aid Effectiveness, Debt Relief and Public Finance Response: Evidence from a Panel of HIPC Countries." *Review of World Economics* 143, no. 4, 742–63.

Cazemajor, Philippe. 1981. *Avocatier, naissance et destruction d'un quartier spontané d'Abidjan*. Abidjan: Centre ORSTOM de Petit-Bassam.

Chaléard, Jean-Louis, and Alain Dubresson. 1989. "Un pied dedans, un pied dehors: À propos du rural et de l'urbain en Côte-d'Ivoire." *Tropiques: Lieux et liens*, Benoît Anthéaume et al., eds., 277–90. Paris: Éditions de l'ORSTOM.

Challenor, Herschelle Sullivan. 1979. "Strangers as Colonial Intermediaries: The Dahomeyans in Francophone Africa." *Strangers in African Societies*, William Shack and Elliot Skinner, eds., 67–83. Berkeley: University of California Press.

Chauveau, Jean-Pierre. 1987. "La part baoulé: Effectif de population et domination ethnique: Une perspective historique." *Cahiers d'études africaines* 27, nos. 105–6, 123–65.

———. 2000. "Question foncière et construction nationale en Côte-d'Ivoire." *Politique africaine* 78, 94–125.

Chauveau, Jean-Pierre, and Jean-Pierre Dozon. 1987. "Au coeur des ethnies ivoiriennes . . . l'état." *L'État contemporain en Afrique*, ed. Emmanuel Terray, 221–96. Paris: l'Harmattan.

Cheater, Angela. 1999. *The Anthropology of Power: Empowerment and Disempowerment in Changing Structures*. London: Routledge.

Chossudovsky, Michel. 1997. *The Globalization of Poverty and the New World Order*. London: Zed Books.

Clastres, Pierre. 1982. *La société contre l'État*. Paris: Éditions de Minuit.

Clignet, Rémi. 1966. "Urbanization and Family Structure in the Ivory Coast." *Comparative Studies in Society and History* 8, no. 4, 385–401.

———. 1967. "Ethnicity, Social Differentiation, and Secondary Schooling in West Africa." *Cahiers d'études africaines* 7, no. 26, 360–78.

Clignet, Rémi, and Philip Foster. 1966. *The Fortunate Few: A Study of Secondary Schools and Students in the Ivory Coast*. Evanston: Northwestern University Press.

Cohen, Michael A. 1972. "The Sans-Travail Demonstrations: The Politics of Frustration in the Ivory Coast." *Manpower and Unemployment Research in Africa* 5, no. 1, 22–25.

———. 1973. "The Myth of the Expanding Centre: Politics in the Ivory Coast." *Journal of Modern African Studies* 11, 227–46.

———. 1974. "Urban Policy and the Decline of the Machine: Cross-Ethnic Politics in the Ivory Coast." *Journal of Developing Areas* 8, no. 2, 227–33.

Cohen, Roger. 2006. "Iraq's Biggest Failing: There Is No Iraq." *New York Times*, 10 December.

Cohen, William B. 1971. *Rulers of Empire: The French Colonial Service in Africa*. Stanford: Hoover Institution Press.

Comaroff, Jean. 2007. "Beyond Bare Life: AIDS, (Bio)politics, and the Neoliberal Order." *Public Culture* 19, no. 1, 197–219.

Conklin, Alice L. 1997. "'Democracy' Rediscovered: Civilization through Association in French West Africa (1914–1930)." *Cahiers d'études africaines* 37, no. 145, 59–84.

———. 1998. "Redefining 'Frenchness': Citizenship, Race Regeneration, and Imperial Motherhood in France and West Africa, 1914–1940." *Domesticating the Empire: Race, Gender and Family Life in French and Dutch Colonialism*, Julia A. Clancy-Smith and France Gouda, eds., 65–83. Charlottesville: University of Virginia Press.

Connelly, Matthew. 2008. *Fatal Misconception: The Struggle to Control World Population*. Cambridge, Mass.: Harvard University Press.

Conrad, Peter, and Joseph Schneider. 1980. "Looking at Levels of Medicalization: A Comment on Strong's Critique of the Thesis of Medical Imperialism." *Social Science and Medicine* 14A, 75–79.

Cooper, Donald B., and Kenneth P. Kiple. 1993. "Yellow Fever." *The Cambridge World History of Human Disease*, ed. Kenneth P. Kiple, 1100–1108. Cambridge: Cambridge University Press.

Cooper, Frederick. 1983. "Urban Space, Industrial Time, and Wage Labor in Africa." *Struggles for the City*, ed. Frederick Cooper, 1–50. London: Sage.

———. 1994. "Conflict and Connection: Rethinking Colonial African History." *American Historical Review* 99 (December), 1516–45.

Cooper, Frederick, and Randall Packard, eds. 1997. *International Development and the Social Sciences*. Berkeley: University of California Press.

Coquery-Vidrovitch, Catherine. 1991. "The Process of Urbanization in Africa (from the Origins to the Beginning of Independence)." *African Studies Review* 34, no. 1, 1–98.

———, ed. 1992. *L'Afrique occidentale au temps des français: Colonisateurs et colonisés, c. 1860–1960*. Paris: Éditions de la découverte.

Cordell, Dennis, Joel Gregory, and Victor Piché. 1996. *Hoe and Wage: A Social History of a Circular Migration System in West Africa*. Boulder: Westview Press.

Coriat, Benjamin. 2008. *The Political Economy of HIV/AIDS in Developing Countries: TRIPS, Public Health Systems and Free Access*. Cheltenham: Edward Elgar Publishing.

Crimp, Douglas. 1988. *AIDS: Cultural Analysis/Cultural Criticism*. Cambridge, Mass.: MIT Press.

Crook, Richard C. 1997. "Winning Coalitions and Ethno-regional Politics: The Failure of the Opposition in the 1990 and 1995 Elections in Côte-d'Ivoire." *African Affairs* 96, 215–42.

Crowder, Michael. 1964. "Indirect Rule: French and British Style." *Africa* 34, no. 3, 197–205.

Cruikshank, Barbara. 1999. *The Will to Empower: Democratic Citizens and Other Subjects.* Ithaca, N.Y.: Cornell University Press.

Curtin, Philip. 1992. "Medical Knowledge and Urban Planning in Colonial Tropical Africa." *The Social Basis of Health and Healing in Africa*, Steven Feierman and John M. Janzen, eds., 235–55. Berkeley: University of California Press.

Da Silva, José Antunes. 1993. "African Independent Churches: Origin and Development." *Anthropos* 88, 393–402.

Dabis, François, Philippe Msellati, Nicolas Meda, Christiane Wiffens-Ekra, Bruno You, Olivier Manigart, Valériane Leroy et al., for the DITRAME Study Group. 1999. "Six-Month Efficacy, Tolerance, and Acceptability of a Short Regimen of Oral Zidovudine to Reduce Vertical Transmission of HIV in Breastfed Children in Côte-d'Ivoire and Burkina Faso: A Double-Blind Placebo-Controlled Multicentre Trial." *Lancet* 353, no. 6, 786–93.

Daddieh, Cyril K. 2001. "Elections and Ethnic Violence in Côte-d'Ivoire: The Unfinished Business of Succession and Democratic Transition." *African Issues* 29, nos. 1–2, 14–19.

Das, Veena, and Ranendra K. Das. 2007. "How the Body Speaks: Illness and the Lifeworld among the Urban Poor." *Subjectivity: Ethnographic Investigations*, Joao Biehl, Byron Good, and Arthur Kleinman, eds., 66–97. Berkeley: University of California Press.

Davis, Mike. 2007. *Planet of Slums.* London: Verso.

De Certeau, Michel. 2002. *The Practice of Everyday Life.* Berkeley: University of California Press.

De Cock, Kevin M. et al. 1989. "Rapid Emergence of AIDS in Abidjan, Ivory Coast." *Lancet* 2, no. 8660, 408–11.

———. 1990. "AIDS: The Leading Cause of Adult Death in the West African City of Abidjan, Ivory Coast." *Science* 249, no. 4970, 793–96.

De Cock, Kevin M., Bernard Barrere, Marie-France Lafontaine, Lacina Diaby, Emmanuel Gnaore, Daniel Pantobe, and Koudou Odehouri. 1991. "Mortality Trends in Abidjan, Côte-d'Ivoire." *AIDS* 5, no. 4, 393–98.

De Miras, Claude. 1980. "Le secteur de subsistence dans les branches de production à Abidjan." *Revue Tiers-Monde* 21, no. 82, 354–72.

Depret, Roland, and Hervé Cames, eds. 1969. "Abidjan-Côte-d'Ivoire: Numéro spécial." *Urbanisme français* 111–12, 1–130.

Derrick, Jonathan. 1983. "The 'Native Clerk' in Colonial West Africa." *Journal of African Affairs* 82, no. 326, 61–74.

Deville-Danthu, Bernadette. 1992. "Les premières tentatives d'encadrement des activités physiques et sportives de la jeunesse en A.O.F. (1922–1936)." *Les jeunes en Afrique, tome 2: La politique et la ville*, Hélène d'Almeida-Torpor, Catherine Coquery-Vidrovitch, Odile Goerg, and Françoise Guitard, eds., 448–62. Paris: l'Harmattan.

Diabaté, Henriette. n.d. *Notre Abidjan.* Abidjan: Mairie d'Abidjan et Ivoire media.

Domergues-Cloarec, Danielle. 1986. *Histoire de la santé en Côte-d'Ivoire.* Toulouse: Presses Universitaires du Mirail.

Dorward, David C. 1974. "Ethnography and Administration: A Study of Anglo-Tiv 'Working Misunderstanding.'" *Journal of African History* 15, no. 3, 457–77.

Dory, Daniel. 1984. "Entre la découverte et la domination: Le Lobi (1800–1960): Éléments d'histoire de la géographie coloniale." *Bulletin de l'association des géographes français* 506, 371–82.

———. 1992. "Géographie et colonisation en France durant la troisième république (1870–1940)." *Science and Empires*, ed. Patrick Petitjean, 323–30. Dordrecht: Kluwer.

Dozon, Jean-Pierre. 1985a. *La société bété*. Paris: Karthala and ORSTOM.

———. 1985b. "Quand les pastoriens traquaient la maladie du sommeil." *Sciences sociales et santé* 3, nos. 3–4, 27–56.

———. 1985c. "Les Bété: Une création coloniale." *Au coeur de l'éthnie: Éthnie, tribalisme et état en Afrique*, Jean-Loup Amselle and Elikia M'Bokolo, eds., 49–86. Paris: Karthala.

———. 1987. "À propos de l'ouvrage de Danielle Comergue-Cloarec: La santé en Côte d'Ivoire 1905–1958." *Psychopathologie Africaine* 21, no. 2, 211–17.

———. 1991. D'un tombeau l'autre. *Cahiers d'études africaines* 31, nos. 121–22, 135–57.

———. 1995. *La cause des prophètes: Politique et religion en Afrique contemporaine*. Paris: Seuil.

———. 1997. "L'étranger et l'allochtone en Côte-d'Ivoire." *Le modèle ivoirien en questions: Crises, ajustements, recompositions*, Bernard Contamin and Harris Memel-Fotê, eds., 779–98. Paris: Karthala and ORSTOM.

———. 2000. "La Côte-d'Ivoire entre démocratie, nationalisme et ethnonationalisme." *Politique africaine* 78, 46–62.

Dubresson, Alain, and Alphonse Yapi-Diahou. 1988. "L'État, 'le bas,' les cours: Exclusion sociale et petite production immobilière à Abidjan (Côte-d'Ivoire)." *Revue Tiers-Monde* 29, no. 116, 1083–1100.

Duranson, Sébastien. 1994. *Impact de la dévaluation du franc CFA sur la filière médicament en Côte d'Ivoire*. Abidjan: Centre ORSTOM de Petit-Bassam.

Dureau, François. 1985. "Migration et urbanisation: Le cas de la Côte-d'Ivoire." PhD diss., Université Paris X—Nanterre.

Duruflé, Gilles. 1988. *L'ajustement structurel en Afrique (Sénégal, Côte-d'Ivoire, Madagascar)*. Paris: Karthala.

Echenberg, Myron J. 1994. "'Faire du Negre': Military Aspects of Population Planning in French West Africa, 1920–1940." *African Population and Capitalism: Historical Perspectives*, Dennis D. Cordell and Joel W. Gregory, eds., 95–108. Madison: University of Wisconsin Press.

———. 2007. *Plague Ports: The Global Urban Impact of Bubonic Plague, 1894–1901*. New York: New York University Press.

Ekeh, Peter P. 1990. "Social Anthropology and Two Contrasting Uses of Tribalism in Africa." *Comparative Studies in Society and History* 32, 660–700.

Elyachar, Julia. 2005. *Markets of Dispossession: NGOs, Economic Development, and the State in Cairo*. Durham, N.C.: Duke University Press.

Epprecht, Marc. 2008. *Heterosexual Africa? The History of an Idea from the Age of Exploration to the Age of AIDS*. Athens: Ohio University Press.

Epstein, Arnold L. 1961. "The Network and Urban Social Organization." *Rhodes-Livingston Institute Journal* 29, 29–61.

———. 1967. "Urbanization and Social Change in Africa." *Current Anthropology* 8, 275–96.

Epstein, Helen. 2008. *The Invisible Cure: Why We Are Losing the Fight against AIDS in Africa*. New York: Farrar, Straus and Giroux.

Epstein, Steve. 1996. *Impure Science: AIDS, Activism, and the Politics of Knowledge*. Berkeley: University of California Press.

Eron, Joseph J. 2008. "Managing Antiretroviral Therapy: Changing Regimens, Resistance Testing, and the Risks from Structured Treatment Interruptions." *Journal of Infectious Diseases* 197, S261–71.

Escobar, Arturo. 1995. *Encountering Development: The Making and Unmaking of the Third World*. Princeton: Princeton University Press.

Étienne, Mona. 1979. "Maternité sociale, rapports d'adoption et pouvoir des femmes chez les Baoulé (Côte-d'Ivoire)." *L'Homme* 19, nos. 3–4, 63–107.

Étienne, Pierre, and Mona Étienne. 1968. "L'émigration Baoulé actuelle." *Cahiers d'outre-mer* 21, no. 82, 155–95.

Eyben, Rosalind. 2000. "Development and Anthropology: A View from Inside the Agency." *Critique of Anthropology* 20, no. 1, 7–14.

Farmer, Paul. 1992. *AIDS and Accusation: Haiti and the Geography of Blame*. Berkeley: University of California Press.

———. 2004a. *Infections and Inequalities: The Modern Plagues*. Berkeley: University of California Press.

———. 2004b. *Pathologies of Power: Health, Human Rights and the New War on the Poor*. Berkeley: University of California Press.

Fassin, Didier. 2001. "The Biopolitics of Otherness: Undocumented Foreigners and Racial Discrimination in French Political Debate." *Anthropology Today* 17, no. 1, 3–7.

———. 2007. *When Bodies Remember: Politics and Experiences of AIDS in South Africa*. Berkeley: University of California Press.

Faubion, James D. 1996. "Kinship Is Dead: Long Live Kinship: A Review Article." *Comparative Studies in Society and History* 38, no. 1, 67–91.

Fauré, Yves A. 1989. "Côte-d'Ivoire: Analyzing the Crisis." *Contemporary West African States*, Donal B. Cruise O'Brien, John Dunn, and Richard Rathbone, eds., 59–74. Cambridge: Cambridge University Press.

Fauré, Yves A., and Jean-François Médard. 1982. "Classe dominante ou classe dirigeante?" *État et bourgeoisie en Côte-d'Ivoire*, Yves A. Fauré and Jean-François Médard, eds., 125–48. Paris: Éditions Karthala.

Ferguson, James. 1994. *The Anti-politics Machine: "Development," Depoliticization, and Bureaucratic Power in Lesotho*. 2nd edn. Minneapolis: University of Minnesota Press.

————. 1999. *Expectations of Modernity: Myths and Meanings of Urban Life on the Zambian Copperbelt*. Berkeley: University of California Press.

Fetter, Bruce. 1987. "Decoding and Interpreting African Census Data: Vital Evidence from an Unsavory Witness." *Cahiers d'études africaines* 27, nos. 105–6, 83–105.

Fink, Sheri. 2009. "Strained by Katrina, a Hospital Faced Deadly Choice." *New York Times*, 25 August 2009.

Fisher, William F. 1997. "Doing Good? The Politics and Antipolitics of NGO Practices." *Annual Reviews of Anthropology* 26, 439–64.

Foller, Maj-Lis, and Hakan Thorn. 2008. *The Politics of AIDS: Globalization, the State and Civil Society*. Basingstoke: Palgrave Macmillan.

Fortes, Meyer. 2008. *African Political Systems*. London: Hesperides Press.

Foster-Carter, Aidan. 1978. "The Modes of Production Controversy." *New Left Review* 107, 47–78.

Foucault, Michel. 1978. *The Will to Knowledge*. Vol. 1 of *The History of Sexuality*. London: Penguin.

————— 1985. *The History of Sexuality, Vol. 2: The Use of Pleasure*. New York: Pantheon Books.

————. 1997a. "Christianity and Confession." *The Politics of Truth*, Sylvère Lotringer and Lysa Hochroth, eds., 199–236. New York: Semiotext.

————. 1997b. "Subjectivity and Truth." *The Politics of Truth*, Sylvère Lotringer and Lysa Hochroth, eds., 171–98. New York: Semiotext.

————. 1998. "Technologies of the Self." *Technologies of the Self*, Luther Martin, Huck Gutman, and Patrick H. Hutton, eds., 16–49. Amherst: University of Massachusetts Press.

Fox, Robin. 1967. *Kinship and Marriage: An Anthropological Perspective*. Cambridge: Cambridge University Press.

Fréchou, Hubert. 1955. "Les plantations européennes en Côte d'Ivoire." *Cahiers d'outre-mer* 8, no. 1, 56–83.

Frenkel, Stephen, and John Western. 1988. "Pretext or Prophylaxis? Racial Segregation and Malarial Mosquitos in a British Tropical Colony: Sierra Leone." *Annals of the Association of American Geographers* 78, no. 2, 211–28.

Gardiner, David. 1985. "The French Impact on Education in Africa, 1817–1960." *Double Impact: France and Africa in the Age of Imperialism*, ed. G. Wesley Johnson 333–44. Westport: Greenwood Press.

Gardner, Katy, and David Lewis. 1995. *Anthropology, Development and the Post-Modern Challenge*. London: Pluto Press.

Garner, Robert C. 2000. "Safe Sects: Dynamic Religion and AIDS in South Africa." *Journal of Modern African Studies* 38, no. 1, 41–69.

Garrett, Laurie. 2007. "The Challenge of Global Health." *Foreign Affairs* 86, no. 1, 14–38.

Gastellu, J. M., and S. Affou Yapi. 1982. "Un mythe à décomposer: La 'bourgeoisie de planteurs.'" *État et bourgeoisie en Côte d'Ivoire*, Yves A. Fauré and Jean-François Médard, eds., 149–80. Paris: Karthala.

Geschiere, Peter, and Reini Raatgever. 1985. "Introduction: Emerging Insights and Issues in French Marxist Anthropology." *Old Modes of Production and Capitalist Encroachment: Anthropological Explorations in Africa*, Wim M. J. van Binsbergen and Peter Geschiere, eds., 1–38. London: KPI.

Gibbal, Jean-Marie. 1974. "La magie à l'école." *Cahiers d'études africaines* 14, no. 56, 627–50.

Gibbal, Jean-Marie, Émile Le Bris, Alain Marie, Annik Osmont, and Gérard Salem. 1982. "Position de l'enquête anthropologique en milieu urbain africain." *Cahiers d'études africaines* 21, nos. 81–83, 7–10.

Ginoux-Pouyaud, Corinne. 1996. "Trajectoires sexuelles et amoureuses: L'exemples des femmes de Marcory et Koumassi (Abidjan)." PhD diss., Université Paul Valéry—Montpellier 3.

Gluckman, Max. 1940. "Analysis of a Social Situation." *Bantu Studies* 14, 147–74.

Gnahoré, Faustin D. 1992. "Recherche sur une expression des jeunes: Le rythme aloucou." *Les jeunes en Afrique: La politique et la ville*, Hélène d'Almeida-Topor, Catherine Coquery-Vidrovitch, Odile Goerg, and Françoise Guitart, eds., 488–520. Paris: Éditions l'Harmattan.

Godelier, Maurice. 1975. "Modes of Production, Kinship, and Demographic Structures." *Marxist Analysis and Social Anthropology*, ed. Maurice Bloch, 3–28. London: Malaby Press.

———. 1978. "Infrastructures, Societies and Histories." *New Left Review* 112, 84–96.

Goldie, Sue J., Yazdan Yazdanpanah, Elena Losina, Milton C. Weinstein, Xavier Anglaret, Rochelle P. Walensky, Heather E. Hsu et al. 2006. "Cost-Effectiveness of HIV Treatment in Resource-Poor Settings: The Case of Côte d'Ivoire." *New England Journal of Medicine* 355, 1141–53.

Gould, Peter. 1993. *The Slow Plague: A Geography of the AIDS Pandemic*. London: Basil Blackwell.

Groff, David H. 1987. "Carrots, Sticks and Cocoa Pods: African and Administrative Initiatives in the Spread of Cocoa Cultivation in Assikasso, Ivory Coast, 1908–1920." *International Journal of African Historical Studies* 20, no. 3, 401–16.

Grootaert, Christiaan, and Ravi Kanbur. 1995. "The Lucky Few amidst Economic Decline: Distributional Change in Côte d'Ivoire as Seen through Panel Data Sets, 1985–1988." *Journal of Development Studies* 31, no. 4, 603–19.

Grootaert, Christiaan, Ravi Kanbur, and Gi-Taik Oh. 1997. "The Dynamics of Welfare Gains and Losses: An African Case Study." *Journal of Development Studies* 33, no. 5, 635–57.

Gruénais, Marc-Éric. 1984. "Dynamiques lignagères et pouvoir en pays Mossi (Burkina Faso)." *Journal des Africanistes* 54, no. 2, 53–74.

Gruskin, Sofia, Katarina Tomasevski, and Aart Hendriks. 1996. "Human Rights and Responses to HIV/AIDS." *AIDS in the World 2*, Jonathan M. Mann and Daniel Tarantola, eds., 326–41. Oxford: Oxford University Press.

Hacking, Ian. 1986. "Making Up People." *Reconstructing Individualism: Autonomy, Indi-*

viduality, and the Self in Western Thought, Thomas C. Heller, Morton Sosna, Christine Brooke-Rose, and David E. Wellbery, eds., 222–36. Palo Alto: Stanford University Press.

———. 1999. *The Social Construction of What?* Cambridge, Mass.: Harvard University Press.

Haeringer, Philippe. 1969a. "Quitte ou double: Les chances de l'agglomération abidjanaise." *Urbanisme français* 111–12, 89–93.

———. 1969b. "Structures foncières et création urbaine à Abidjan." *Cahiers d'études africaines* 9, no. 34, 219–70.

———. 1988. "L'explosion de l'offre artisanale à Abidjan et ses relations avec la récession économique (1980–1985)." *Espace, Populations, Sociétés* 2, 275–94.

Hannaway, Caroline. 1993. "Environment and Miasmata." *Companion Encyclopedia of the History of Medicine*, Roy Porter and William F. Bynum, eds., 292–308. London: Routledge.

Hansen, Karen Tranberg. 2004. "Who Rules the Streets? The Politics of Vending Space in Lusaka." *Reconsidering Informality: Perspectives from Urban Africa*, Karen T. Hansen and Mariken Vaa, eds., 62–80. Uppsala: Nordic Africa Institute.

Hart, Keith. 1973. "Informal Income Opportunities and Urban Employment in Ghana." *Journal of Modern African Studies* 11, no. 1, 61–89.

Harvey, David. 1994. *The Postmodern Condition*. London: Basil Blackwell.

———. 2005. *A Brief History of Neoliberalism*. Oxford: Oxford University Press.

Hawkin, Kirstan, N. Price, and Fatima Mussa. 2009. "Milking the Cow: Young Women's Construction of Identity and Risk in Age-Disparate Transactional Sexual Relationships in Maputo, Mozambique." *Global Public Health* 4, no. 2, 169–82.

Hays, J. N. 1998. *The Burdens of Disease: Epidemics and Human Response in Western History*. New Brunswick, N.J.: Rutgers University Press.

Heath, Deborah, Rayna Rapp, and Karen-Sue Taussig. 2004. "Genetic Citizenship." *Companion to the Anthropology of Politics*, David Nugent and Joan Vincent, eds., 152–67. Oxford: Blackwell.

Hecht, Robert M. 1984. "The Transformation of Lineage Production in Southern Ivory Coast, 1920–1980." *Ethnology* 23, no. 4, 261–78.

Hellweg, Joseph. 2004. "Encompassing the State." *Africa Today* 50, no. 4, 3–28.

———. 2009. "Hunters, Ritual and Freedom: Sozo Sacrifice as a Technology of the Self in the Benkadi Movement of Côte d'Ivoire." *Journal of the Royal Anthropological Institute* 15, 36–56.

Hoad, Neville. 2007. *African Intimacies: Race, Homosexuality and Globalization*. Minneapolis: University of Minnesota Press.

Holas, Bohumil. 1954. "Bref aperçu sur les principaux cultes syncrétiques de la Basse-Côte-d'Ivoire." *Africa* 24, no. 1, 55–60.

Hunt, Nancy Rose. 1994. "Letter-Writing, Nursing Men, and Bicycles in the Belgian Congo: Notes towards the Social Identity of a Colonial Category." *Paths towards the*

Past: African Historical Essays in Honor of Jan Vansina, Robert W. Harms et al., eds., 187–210. Atlanta: African Studies Association Press.

———. 1997. "Condoms, Confessors, Conferences: Among AIDS Derivatives in Africa." *Journal of the International Institute* 4, no. 3. Available online from the web site of the *Journal of the International Institute* at the University of Michigan.

———. 1999. *A Colonial Lexicon of Birth Ritual, Medicalization, and Mobility in the Congo*. Durham, N.C.: Duke University Press.

Hunter, Mark. 2002. "The Materiality of Everyday Sex: Thinking beyond 'Prostitution.'" *African Studies* 61, no. 1, 99–120.

———. 2006. "The Changing Political Economy of Sex in South Africa: The Significance of Unemployment and Inequalities to the Scale of the AIDS Pandemic." *Social Science and Medicine* 64, no. 3, 689–700.

Huysmans, Jef. 2004. "Minding Exceptions: The Politics of Insecurity and Liberal Democracy." *Contemporary Political Theory* 3, no. 3, 321–41.

Institut National de la Statistique (INS), Ministère de la Lutte contre le Sida [Côte d'Ivoire], and ORC Macro. 2006. *Enquête sur les indicateurs du Sida, Côte d'Ivoire 2005*. Calverton, Md.: INS and ORC Macro.

Institute of Medicine, Board on Population Health and Public Health Practice. 2005. *Review of the HIVNET 012 Perinatal HIV Prevention Study*. Washington: National Academies Press.

International Labour Office. 1972. *Incomes, Employment and Equality in Kenya*. Geneva: International Labour Office.

Iverson, Kenneth V., and John C. Moskop. 2007. "Triage in Medicine, Part 1: Concept, History and Types." *Annals of Emergency Medicine* 49, no. 3, 282–87.

Janzen, John. 1982. *The Quest for Therapy: Medical Pluralism in Lower Zaïre*. Berkeley: University of California Press.

Jarret, Marie-France, and François Régis Mahieu. 1991. "Ajustement structurel, croissance et répartition: L'exemple de la Côte-d'Ivoire." *Revue Tiers Monde* 32, no. 125, 39–62.

Jézéquel, Jean-Hervé. 1999. "Le 'théâtre des instituteurs' en Afrique Occidentale française (1930–1950): Pratique socio-culturelle et vecteur de cristallisation de nouvelles identités urbaines." *Fêtes urbaines en Afrique*, ed. Odile Goerg, 182–200. Paris: Karthala.

Jones, James H. 1993. *Bad Blood: The Tuskegee Syphilis Experiment*. Rev. edn. New York: Free Press.

Joshi, Heather, Harold Lubell, and Jean Mouly. 1976. *Abidjan: Urban Development and Employment in the Ivory Coast*. Geneva: International Labour Office.

Kaddar, Miloud, and Eliane Furrer. 2008. "Are Current Debt Relief Initiatives an Option for Scaling up Health Financing in Beneficiary Countries?" *Bulletin of the World Health Organization* 86, no. 11, 817–908.

Kadet, G. Bertin. 1999. "Urbanisation et pauvreté: Aspects de la condition citadine dans la région des montagnes, en Côte-d'Ivoire." *Cahiers d'outre-mer* 52, no. 206, 197–218.

Kalofonos, Ippolytos. 2008. "A Vida Positiva: Activism, Evangelism and Antiretrovirals in Mozambique." PhD diss., University of California, San Francisco.

Kanbur, Ravi. 1990. *Poverty and the Social Dimensions of Structural Adjustment in Côte-d'Ivoire*. Washington: World Bank.

Kayal, Philip M. 1993. *Bearing Witness: Gay Men's Health Crisis and the Politics of AIDS*. Boulder: Westview Press.

Kieffer, Guy-André. 2000. "Armée ivoirienne: Le refus ou déclassement." *Politique africaine* 78, 26–44.

Kipré, Pierre. 1988. "Sociétés urbaines africaines et pratiques sociales de l'espace urbain: Le cas ivoirien (1930–1960)." *Processus d'urbanisation en Afrique*, ed. Catherine Coquery-Vidrovitch, 37–45. Paris: Karthala.

Kirschke, Linda. 2000. "Informal Repression: Zero-Sum Politics and Late Third Wave Transitions." *Journal of Modern African Studies* 38, no. 3, 383–405.

Kouakou N'Guessan, François. 1983. "Les 'maquis' d'Abidjan: Nourritures du terroir et fraternité citadine, ou la conscience de classe autour d'un foutou d'igname." *Cahiers ORSTOM, série sciences humaines* 19, no. 4, 545–50.

Kramer, Jane. 1993. "Letter from Europe: Bad Blood." *New Yorker*, 11 October, 74–95.

Laga, Marie, Bernhard Schwartlander, Elisabeth Pisani, Papa Salif Sow, and Michel Carael. 2001. "To Stem HIV in Africa, Prevent Transmission to Young Women." *AIDS* 15, 931–34.

Latour, Bruno. 1986. "Le théâtre de la preuve." *Pasteur et la Révolution Pastorienne*, ed. Claire Salomon-Bayet, 335–84. Paris: Payot.

———. 1988. *The Pasteurization of France*. Cambridge, Mass.: Harvard University Press.

Laurent, Pierre-Joseph. 1998. "Conversions aux assemblées de Dieu chez les Mossi du Burkina Faso: 'Modernité et sociabilité.'" *Journal des Africanistes* 68, nos. 1–2, 67–97.

Le Pape, Marc. 1985. "De l'espace et des races à Abidjan, entre 1903 et 1934." *Cahiers d'études africaines* 25, no. 99, 295–307.

———. 1986. "Les statuts d'une génération: Les déscolarisés d'Abidjan entre 1976 et 1986." *Politique africaine* 29, 104–12.

———. 1997. *L'Énergie sociale à Abidjan: Économie politique de la ville en Afrique noire, 1930–1995*. Paris: Karthala.

Le Pape, Marc, and Claudine Vidal. 1982. "Raisons pratiques africaines." *Cahiers internationaux de sociologie* 73, 293–321.

———. 1984. "Libéralisme et vécus sexuels à Abidjan." *Cahiers internationaux de sociologie* 16, 111–18.

———. 1987. "L'école à tout prix: Stratégies éducatives dans la petite bourgeoisie d'Abidjan." *Actes de la recherche en sciences sociales* 70, 64–73.

———. 2002. *Côte-d'Ivoire: L'année terrible (1999–2000)*. Paris: Karthala.

Le Pape, Marc, Claudine Vidal, and Alphonse Yapi-Diahou. 1991. "Abidjan: Du cosmopolitisme à la mondialisation." *Métropoles du tiers monde—ASP ORSTOM—CNRS*. Unpublished typescript.

Leclerc-Madlala, Suzanne. 2003. "Transactional Sex and the Pursuit of Modernity." *Social Dynamics* 29, 213–33.

Lee, Laura Kim. 2002. "Changing Selves, Changing Society: Human Relations Experts and the Invention of T Groups, Sensitivity Training and Encounter in the United States, 1938–1980." PhD diss., University of California, Los Angeles.

Lefebvre, Henri. 1991. *The Production of Space*. London: Blackwell Publishing.

———. 1995. *Writings on Cities*. London: Blackwell Publishing.

Li, Tania M. 2007. *The Will to Improve: Governmentality, Development and the Practice of Politics*. Durham, N.C.: Duke University Press.

Lindenbaum, Shirley, and Gilbert Herdt. 1992. *The Time of AIDS: Social Analysis, Theory, and Method*. London: Sage Publications.

Lindenbaum, Shirley, and Margaret Lock, eds. 1993. *Knowledge, Power and Practice: The Anthropology of Medicine and Everyday Life*. Berkeley: University of California Press.

Little, Kenneth. 1962. "Some Traditionally Based Forms of Mutual Aid in West African Urbanization." *Ethnology* 1, no. 2, 197–211.

Lock, Margaret, and Deborah R. Gordon, eds. 1988. *Biomedicine Examined*. Dordrecht: Kluwer Academic Publishers.

Lock, Margaret, and Patricia A. Kaufert. 1998a. "Introduction." *Pragmatic Women and Body Politics*, Margaret Lock and Patricia A. Kaufert, eds., 1–27. Cambridge: Cambridge University Press.

———, eds. 1998b. *Pragmatic Women and Body Politics*. Cambridge: Cambridge University Press.

Lohse, Nicolai, Ann-Brit Eg Hansen, Gitte Pedersen, Gitte Kronborg, Jan Gerstoft, Henrik Toft Sørensen, Michael Væth, and Niels Obel. 2007. "Survival of Persons with and without HIV Infection in Denmark, 1995–2005." *Annals of Internal Medicine* 146, no. 2, 87–95.

Losch, Bruno. 2000. "La Côte-d'Ivoire en quête d'un nouveau projet national." *Politique africaine* 78, 5–21.

Losina, Elena, Yazdan Yazdanpanah, Sylvie Deuffic-Burban, Bingxia Wang, Lindsey L. Wolf, Eugène Messou, Delphine Gabillard, Catherine Seyler, Kenneth A. Freedberg, and Xavier Anglaret. 2007. "The Independent Effect of Highly Active Antiretroviral Therapy on Severe Opportunistic Disease Incidence and Mortality in HIV-Infected Adults in Cote d'Ivoire." *Antivir Ther* 12, no. 4, 543–51.

Luke, Nancy. 2003. "Age and Economic Asymmetries in the Sexual Relationships of Adolescent Girls in Sub-Saharan Africa." *Studies in Family Planning* 34, 67–86.

Maganja, R. K., S. Maman, A. Groves, and J. K. Mbwambo. 2007. "Skinning the Goat and Pulling the Load: Transactional Sex among Youth in Dar es Salaam, Tanzania." *AIDS Care* 19, no. 8, 974–81.

Magubane, Bernard. 1971. "A Critical Look at the Indices Used in the Study of Social Change in Colonial Africa." *Current Anthropology* 12, nos. 4–5, 419–55.

Mahieu, François Régis. 1995. "Variable Dimension in the Côte-d'Ivoire: Reasons for Failure." *Review of African Political Economy* 22, no. 63, 9–26.

Mamdani, Mahmood. 1996. *Citizen and Subject: Contemporary Africa and the Legacy of Late Colonialism.* Princeton: Princeton University Press.

———. 2001. "Beyond Settler and Native as Political Identities: Overcoming the Political Legacy of Colonialism." *Comparative Studies in Society and History* 43, no. 4, 651–64.

Mann, Jonathan, and Daniel Tarantola. 1996. *AIDS in the World 2.* Oxford: Oxford University Press.

Manou-Savina, Annie. 1985. "Politiques et pratiques urbaines à Abidjan." PhD diss., Université de Paris 1.

———. 1989. "Éléments pour une histoire de la cour commune en milieu urbain: Réflexions sur le cas ivoirien." *Tropiques: Lieux et liens*, Benoît Anthéaume et al., eds., 310–17. Paris: Éditions de l'ORSTOM.

Manou-Savina, Annie, and Alain Dubresson. 1985. "Abidjan-populaire: Au-delà des apparences." *Cités africaines* 2, 19–50.

Marais, Hein. 2005. "Buckling: The Impact of AIDS on South Africa." Pretoria: Centre for the Study of AIDS. PDF available from the web site of the Centre for the Study of AIDS, www.csa.za.org.

Marcovich, Anne. 1988. "French Colonial Medicine and Colonial Rule: Algeria and Indochina." *Disease, Medicine, and Empire: Perspectives on Western Medicine and the Experience of European Expansion*, Roy M. MacLeod and Milton James Lewis, eds., 103–20. London: Taylor and Francis.

Marguerat, Yves. 1998. "L'étude des violences urbaines d'Ibadan (1994) à Abidjan (1997)." *Cahiers d'études africaines* 38, nos. 150–2, 665–71.

Marie, Alain. 1997a. "Du sujet communautaire au sujet individuel: Une lecture anthropologique de la réalité africaine contemporaine." *L'Afrique des individus*, ed. Alain Marie, 53–112. Paris: Karthala.

———. 1997b. "Avatars de la dette communautaire: Crise des solidarités, sorcellerie et procès d'individualisation (itinéraires abidjanais)." *L'Afrique des individus*, ed. Alain Marie, 249–330. Paris: Karthala.

Martin, Emilie. 1995. *Flexible Bodies: The Role of Immunity in American Culture from the Days of Polio to the Age of AIDS.* Boston: Beacon.

Martin, Guy. 1995. "Continuity and Change in Franco-African Relations." *Journal of Modern African Studies* 33, no. 1, 1–20.

Martin, Michèle. 2003. *"Hello Central?": Gender, Technology, and Culture in the Formation of Telephone Systems.* Montréal: McGill-Queen's University Press.

Martin, Phyllis. 1985. *Leisure and Society in Colonial Brazzaville.* Cambridge: Cambridge University Press.

Mary, André. 1997. "La tradition prophétique ivoirienne au regard de l'histoire." *Cahiers d'études africaines* 37, no. 145, 213–23.

———. 1999. "Culture pentecôtiste et charisme visionnaire au sein d'une église indépendante africaine." *Archives de sciences sociales des religions* 105, 29–50.

Mbembe, Achille. 2002. "African Modes of Self-Writing." *Public Culture* 14, no. 1, 239–73.

McFalls, Laurence. 2007. "A Matter of Life and Death: Iatrogenic Violence and the

Formal Logic of International Intervention." Working Paper CSGP 07/7. Centre for the Study of Global Power and Politics, Trent University. PDF available from the web site of Centre for the Study of Global Power and Politics.

Middleton, John, and David Tait. 1958. "Introduction." *Tribes without Rulers: Studies in African Segmentary Systems*, John Middleton and David Tait, eds., 1–31. London: Routledge.

Mitchell, J. Clyde. 1956. *The Kalela Dance*. Manchester: Manchester University Press.

Morgan, Henry Lewis. 1877. *Ancient Society: Researches in the Lines of Human Progress from Savagery through Barbarism to Civilization*. New York: Henry Holt and Company.

Moulin, Anne-Marie. 1992. "Patriarchal Science: The Network of the Overseas Pasteur Institutes." *Science and Empires: Historical Studies about Scientific Development and European Expansion*, Patrick Petitjean, Catherine Jami, and Anne Marie Moulin, eds., 307–22. Boston Studies in the Philosophy of Science 136. Dordrecht: Kluwer.

———. 1996. "Tropical without the Tropics: The Turning-Point of Pastorian Medicine in North Africa." *Warm Climates and Western Medicine: The Emergence of Tropical Medicine 1500–1900*, ed. David Arnold, 160–207. Amsterdam: Rodopi.

Msellati, Philippe, Laurent Vidal, and Jean-Paul Moatti, eds. 2001. *L'accès aux traitements du VIH/sida en Côte d'Ivoire: Evaluation de l'initiative, Onusida/ministère ivoirien de la santé publique: Aspects économiques, sociaux et comportementaux*. Coll. sciences sociales et sida. Paris: Agence nationale de recherches sur le sida.

Newell, Sasha. 2006. "Estranged Belongings: A Moral Economy of Theft in Abidjan, Côte-d'Ivoire." *Anthropological Theory* 6, no. 2, 179.

Nguyen, Vinh-Kim. 2002. "Sida, ONG et politique du témoignage." *Anthropologie et sociétés* 26, no. 1, 69–87.

———. 2004. "Antiretroviral Globalism, Biopolitics and Therapeutic Citizenship." *Global Assemblages: Technology, Politics and Ethics*, Aihwa Ong and Stephen Collier, eds., 124–44. London: Blackwell.

———. 2005. "Uses and Pleasures." *Sex in Development: Science, Sexuality, and Morality in Global Perspective*, Stacy L. Pigg and Vincanne Adams, eds., 245–68. Durham, N.C.: Duke University Press.

———. 2009a. "Government-by-Exception: Enrolment and Experimentality in Mass HIV Treatment Programmes in Africa." *Social Theory and Health* 7, no. 3, 196–217.

———. 2009b. "Therapeutic Evangelism: Confessional Technologies, Antiretrovirals, and Biospiritual Transformation in the Fight against AIDS in West Africa." *AIDS and Religious Practice in Africa*, Felicitas Becker and P. Wessler Geissler, eds., 359–78. Leiden: Brill.

Nkengasong, John N., Christiane Adje-Touré, and Paul J. Weidle. 2004. "HIV Antiretroviral Drug Resistance in Africa." *AIDS Rev* 6, 4–12.

Oliveira, Maria A., Elizabeth M. dos Santos, and José M. Mello. 2001. "AIDS, Activism and the Regulation of Clinical Trials in Brazil: Protocol 028." *Cad Saude Publica* 17, no. 4, 863–75.

Olivier de Sardan, Jean-Pierre. 1999. "A Moral Economy of Corruption in Africa?" *Journal of Modern African Studies* 37, no. 1, 25–52.

———. 2005. *Anthropology and Development: Understanding Contemporary Social Change*. London: Zed Books.

O'Malley, Jeffrey O., Vinh-Kim Nguyen, and Sarah Lee. 1996. "Non-governmental Organizations." *AIDS in the World 2*, Jonathan M. Mann and Daniel Tarantola, eds., 341–61. London: Oxford University Press.

O'Manique, Colleen. 2004. *Neoliberalism and AIDS Crisis in Sub-Saharan Africa: Globalization's Pandemic*. Basingstoke: Palgrave-Macmillan.

Ong, Aihwa. 2006. *Neoliberalism as Exception: Mutations in Citizenship and Sovereignty*. Berkeley: University of California Press.

Owen, David. 1999. "Power, Knowledge and Ethics: Foucault." *Edinburgh Encyclopedia of Continental Philosophy*, ed. Simon Glendinning, 593–604. London: Routledge.

Packard, Randall M. 1989. "The 'Healthy Reserve' and the 'Dressed Native': Discourses on Black Health and the Language of Legitimation in South Africa." *American Ethnologist* 16, 686–703.

Pakenham, Thomas. 1992. *The Scramble for Africa*. London: Abacus.

Pandolfi, Mariella. 2000. "Une souveraineté mouvante et supracoloniale: L'industrie humanitaire dans les Balkans." *Multitudes* 3, 97–105.

———. 2006. "La zone grise des guerres humanitaires." *Anthropologica* 48, no. 1, 43–58.

———. 2008. "Laboratory of Intervention: The Humanitarian Governance of the Postcommunist Balkan Territories." *Postcolonial Disorders*, Mary-Jo DelVecchio Good, Sandra T. Hyde, and Byron J. Good, eds., 157–88. Berkeley: University of California Press.

Parkin, David. 1966. "Urban Voluntary Associations as Institutions of Adaptation." *Man* 1, no. 1, 90–94.

Patton, Cindy. 1990. *Inventing AIDS*. New York: Routledge.

Paulme, Denise. 1963. "Une religion syncrétique en Côte d'Ivoire: Le culte *deima*." *Cahiers d'études africaines* 3, no. 9, 5–90.

Péducasse, Virginie. 1996. "Sida et confessions à Abidjan: De la Bible au Coran en passant par l'arrêté ministériel portant création du programme national de lutte contre le Sida." Mémoire DEA (Master's thesis), Université de Bordeaux 4.

Peires, Jeffrey B. 1989. *The Dead Will Arise: Nongqawuse and the Great Xhosa Cattle-Killing Movement of 1856-7*. Bloomington: Indiana University Press.

Peletz, Michael G. 1995. "Kinship Studies in Late Twentieth-Century Anthropology." *Annual Review of Anthropology* 24, 343–72.

PEPFAR. 2007. "The Power of Partnerships: The President's Emergency Plan for AIDS Relief." Third Annual Report to Congress. Washington: Office of the Global AIDS Coordinator.

———. 2009. "Making a Difference: Funding." Washington: Office of the Global AIDS Coordinator. www.PEPFAR.gov.

Perkins, John. 2005. *Confessions of an Economic Hit Man*. New York: Plume.

Perrot, Claude-Hélène. 1987. "La sensibilité des sociétés akan du sud-est de la Côte d'Ivoire aux fluctuations démographiques." *Cahiers d'études africaines* 27, nos. 105–6, 167–75.

———. 1996. "Les ravages des prophètes dans les civilisations paysannes." *Journal des Africanistes* 66, nos. 1–2, 319–31.

Peschard, Karine. 2001. "Access to HIV Treatment from a Historical and Social Perspective." Honor's thesis, Department of Anthropology, McGill University.

Petryna, Adriana, 2002. *Life Exposed: Biological Citizens after Chernobyl.* Princeton: Princeton University Press.

———. 2005. "Ethical Variability: Drug Development and Globalizing Clinical Trials." *American Ethnologist* 32, no. 2, 183–97.

———. 2009. *When Experiments Travel: Clinical Trials and the Global Search for Human Subjects.* Princeton: Princeton University Press.

Pfeiffer, James. 2004. "Condom Social Marketing, Pentecostalism, and Structural Adjustment in Mozambique: A Clash of AIDS Prevention Messages. *Medical Anthropology Quarterly* 18, no. 1, 77–103.

Piault, Colette. 1975. *Prophétisme et thérapeutique: Albert Atcho et la communauté de Bregbo.* Paris: Hermann.

Pigg, Stacy Leigh. 2001. "Languages of Sex and AIDS in Nepal: Notes on the Social Production of Commensurability." *Cultural Anthropology* 16, no. 4, 481–541.

———. 2005. "Globalizing the Facts of Life." *Sex in Development: Science, Sexuality, and Morality in Global Perspective*, Vincanne Adams and Stacy Leigh Pigg, eds., 39–65. Durham, N.C.: Duke University Press.

Poku, Nana K., and Alan Whiteside., eds. 2002. "Global Health and Governance: HIV/AIDS." Special issue, *Third World Quarterly* 23, no. 2, 189–350.

Pollak, Michael. 1988. *Les homosexuels et le sida.* Paris: Métailié.

Pompey, Fabienne. 1999. "Joséphine Oupoh a créé une association ivoirienne de femmes séropositives 'pour en parler.'" *Le Monde*, 14 September.

Posel, Deborah. 2008. "History as Confession: The Case of the South African Truth and Reconciliation Commission." *Public Culture* 20, no. 1, 119–41.

Prince, Ruth. 2007. "Salvation and Tradition: Configurations of Faith in a Time of Death." *Journal of Religion in Africa* 37, no. 1, 84–115.

Proteau, Laurence. 1997. "Dévoilement de l'illusion d'une promotion sociale pour tous par l'école: Un 'moment critique.'" *Le modèle ivoirien en questions: Crises, ajustements, recompositions*, Bernard Contamin and Harris Memel-Fotê, eds. 635–54. Paris: Karthala and ORSTOM.

Raatgever, Reini. 1985. "Analytic Tools, Intellectual Weapons: The Discussion among French Marxist Anthropologists about the Identification of Modes of Production in Africa." *Old Modes of Production and Capitalist Encroachment: Anthropological Explorations in Africa*, Wim M. J. van Binsbergen and Peter Geschiere, eds., 290–330. London: KPI.

Rabinow, Paul. 1992. "Artificiality and Enlightenment: From Sociobiology to Biosociality." *Incorporations*, Jonathan Crary and Sanford Kwiner, eds., 234–52. New York: Zone Books.

Radcliffe-Brown, Alfred R., and Daryll Forde. 1950. *African Systems of Kinship and Marriage*. Oxford: Oxford University Press.

Ranger, Terence O. 1986. "Religious Movements and Politics in Sub-Saharan Africa." *African Studies Review* 29, 1–69.

Ranger, Terence, and Paul Slack. 1995. *Epidemics and Ideas: Essays on the Historical Perception of Pestilence*. Cambridge: Cambridge University Press.

Reporters without Borders. 2009. "Five Years of Unanswered Questions since Journalist's Abduction in Abidjan." Available at the web site of Reporters without Borders, www.rsf.org.

Richey, Lisa. 2008. "Better (Red)™ than Dead?: Celebrities, Consumption and International Aid." *Third World Quarterly* 29, no. 4, 711–29.

Riles, Annelise. 2001. *The Network Inside Out*. Ann Arbor: University of Michigan Press.

Robins, Steven L. 2006. "From Rights to 'Ritual': AIDS Activism and Treatment Testimonies in South Africa." *American Anthropologist* 108, no. 2, 312–23.

Rogers, Carl R. 1970. *Carl Rogers on Encounter Groups*. New York: Harper and Row.

Roitman, Janet. 1990. "The Politics of Informal Markets in Sub-Saharan Africa." *Journal of Modern African Studies* 28, no. 4, 671–96.

———. 2004. *Fiscal Disobedience: An Anthropology of Economic Regulation in Central Africa*. Princeton: Princeton University Press.

Rose, Nikolas. 2006. *The Politics of Life Itself: Biomedicine, Power, and Subjectivity in the Twenty-First Century*. Princeton: Princeton University Press.

———. 2007. "Beyond Medicalization." *Lancet* 369, 700–702.

Rose, Nikolas, and Carlos Novas. 2004. "Biological Citizenship." *Global Assemblages: Technology, Politics, and Ethics as Anthropological Problems*, Aihwa Ong and Stephen J. Collier, eds., 439–63. London: Blackwell.

Rosenberg, Charles E. 1992. *Explaining Epidemics*. Cambridge: Cambridge University Press.

Rouch, Jean. 1963. "Introduction à l'étude de la communauté de Bregbo." *Journal des Africanistes* 33, 129–202.

Rouch, Jean, and Edmond Bernus. 1957. "Note sur les prostituées 'toutou' de Treichville et d'Adjamé." *Études éburnéennes* 6, 231–42.

Scheper-Hughes, Nancy. 2003. "Rotten Trade: Millennial Capitalism, Human Values and Global Justice in Organs Trafficking." *Journal of Human Rights* 2, no. 2, 197–226.

Schmitt, Carl. 2005. *Political Theology: Four Chapters on the Concept of Sovereignty*. Chicago: University of Chicago Press.

Schwab, William B. 1970. "Urbanism, Corporate Groups and Culture Change in Africa below the Sahara." *Anthropological Quarterly* 43, no. 3, 187–214.

Scott, Guy. 2000. "Political Will, Political Economy and the AIDS Industry in Zambia." *Review of African Political Economy* 27, no. 86, 577.

Scott, James C. 1976. *The Moral Economy of the Peasant: Rebellion and Subsistence in Southeast Asia*. New Haven: Yale University Press.

Seidel, Gill. 1993. "The Competing Discourses of HIV/AIDS in Sub-Saharan Africa: Discourses of Rights and Empowerment vs. Discourses of Control and Exclusion." *Social Science and Medicine* 36, no. 3, 175–94.

Setel, Philip. 1999. *A Plague of Paradoxes: AIDS, Culture, and Demography in Northern Tanzania*. Chicago: University of Chicago Press.

Shacinda, Shapi. 2005. "Zambia to Put Debt Relief into AIDS Fight." Reuters. Available on Global Exchange, www.globalexchange.org.

Shank, David A. 1994. *Prophet Harris, the 'Black Elijah' of West Africa*, abridged by Jocelyn Murray. Leiden: Brill.

———. 1999. "Le pentecôtisme du prophète William Wadé Harris." *Archives de sciences sociales des religions* 105, 51–70.

Sibeud, Emmanuelle. 1994. "La naissance de l'ethnographie africaniste en France avant 1914." *Cahiers d'études africaines* 34, no. 136, 639–58.

Silberschmidt, Margrethe, and Vibeke Rasch. 2001. "Adolescent Girls, Illegal Abortions and 'Sugar Daddies' in Dar es Salaam: Vulnerable Victim and Active Social Agents." *Social Science and Medicine* 52, 1815–26.

Sirven, Pierre. 1967. "Les conséquences géographiques d'un nouveau syncrétisme religieux en Côte-d'Ivoire: Le Kokambisme." *Cahiers d'outre-mer* 78, 127–36.

Skinner, Elliott P. 1974. *African Urban Life: The Transformation of Ouagadougou*. Princeton: Princeton University Press.

Smith, Daniel Jordan. 2001. "Kinship and Corruption in Contemporary Nigeria." *Ethnos* 66, no. 3, 344–64.

———. 2003. "Patronage, Per Diems and the 'Workshop Mentality': The Practice of Family Planning Programs in Southeastern Nigeria." *World Development* 31, no. 4, 703–15.

———. 2004. "Youth, Sin and Sex in Nigeria: Christianity and HIV/AIDS-related Beliefs and Behaviour among Rural-Urban Migrant." *Culture, Health and Sexuality* 6, no. 5, 425–37.

Sparke, Matthew. 2009. "Unpacking Economism and Remapping the Terrain of Global Health." *Global Health Governance: Crisis, Institutions and Political Economy*, Adrian Kay and Owain D. Williams, eds., 131–59. Basingstoke: Palgrave Macmillan.

Stiglitz, Joseph E. 2003. *Globalization and Its Discontents*. New York: Penguin.

Stirrat, Roderick L. 2000. "Cultures of Consultancy." *Critique of Anthropology* 20, no. 1, 31–46.

Stolberg, Sheryl Gay. 2001. "AIDS Groups Revive a Fight, and Themselves." *New York Times*, 20 March.

Suret-Canale, Jean. 1982. "'Resistance' et 'collaboration' en Afrique noire coloniale." *Études africaines offertes à Henri Brunschwig*, Henri Brunschwig and Jan Vansina, eds., 319–31. Paris: Éditions de l'École des hautes études en sciences sociales.

Swanson, Maynard W. 1977. "The Sanitation Syndrome: Bubonic Plague and Urban Native Policy in the Cape Colony 1900–1909." *Journal of African History* 18, no. 3, 387–410.

Taussig, Michael. 1980. "Reification and the Consciousness of the Patient." *Social Science and Medicine* 14B, no. 1, 3–13.

Taylor, Chloë. 2009. *The Culture of Confession from Augustine to Foucault: A Genealogy of the "Confessing Animal."* New York: Routledge.

Thompson, Edward P. 1971. "The Moral Economy of the English Crowd in the Eighteenth Century." *Past and Present* 50, 76–134.

Thoret, Jean-Claude. 1974. "Les jeunes Djimini: Essai sur la dynamique des groupes de jeunes." PhD diss., Université de Paris, École pratique des hautes études.

Thornton, Robert. 2008. *Unimagined Community: Sex, Networks, and AIDS in Uganda and South Africa*. Berkeley: University of California Press.

Ticktin, Miriam. 2006. "Where Ethics and Politics Meet: The Violence of Humanitarianism in France." *American Ethnologist* 33, no. 1, 33–49.

Tirefort, Alain. 1983. "Un monde policé en terre ivoirienne: Le cercle toubabou, 1904–1939." *Cahiers d'études africaines* 23, nos. 89–90, 97–119.

———. 1992. "Le métissage en Côte-d'Ivoire: 1893–1960." *Les jeunes en Afrique, tome 1: évolution et rôle (XIXe-XXe siècles)*, Hélène d'Almeida-Torpor, Catherine Coquery-Vidrovitch, Odile Goerg, and Françoise Guitard, eds., 83–102. Paris: l'Harmattan.

———. 1999. "Aux antipodes du Tam-tam: La fête coloniale en Côte-d'Ivoire pendant l'entre-deux-guerres." *Fêtes urbaines en Afrique*, ed. Odile Goerg, 167–79. Paris: Karthala.

Touré, Abdou. 1985. *Les petits métiers à Abidjan*. Paris: Karthala.

Treichler, Paula. 1987. "AIDS, Homophobia, and Biomedical Discourse: An Epidemic of Signification." *Cultural Studies* 1, 263–305.

UNAIDS. 2008. "Report on the Global AIDS Epidemic."

Verghese, Abraham. 1995. *My Own Country: A Doctor's Story*. New York: Vintage.

Vidal, Claudine. 1977. "Guerre des sexes à Abidjan: Masculin, féminin, CFA." *Cahiers d'études africaines* 17, no. 65, 121–53.

———. 1979. "L'argent fini, l'amour est envolé . . ." *L'Homme* 19, nos. 3–4, 1–18.

———. 1980. "Pour un portrait d'Abidjan avec dames." *Cahiers internationaux de sociologie* 69, 305–12.

———. 1990. "Abidjan: Quand les 'petits' deviennent des pauvres." *Politique africaine* 39, 166–70.

———. 1991. *Sociologie des passions: Rwanda, Côte d'Ivoire*. Paris: Karthala.

———. 1997. "Du rêve au réalisme: Des citadins sans illusion 1970–1994." *Le modèle ivoirien en questions: Crises, ajustements, recompositions*, Bernard Contamin and Harris Memel-Fotê, eds., 655–68. Paris: Karthala and ORSTOM.

Vimard, Patrice, and Sombo N'Cho. 1995. "Évolution de la structure des ménages et différenciation des modèles familiaux en Côte-d'Ivoire 1975–1993." *Ménages et familles* en Afrique: Approche des dynamiques contemporaines, Marc Pilon, Thérèse Locoh, Émilien Vignikin, and Patrice Vimard, eds., 101–21. Les Études du CEPED, no. 15. Paris: Centre français sur la population et le développement.

Walker, Neff, Nicholas C. Grassly, Geoff P. Garnett, Karen A. Stanecki, and Peter D. Ghys. 2004. "Estimating the Global Burden of HIV/AIDS: What Do We Really Know about the HIV Pandemic?" *Lancet* 363, no. 9427, 2180–85.

Wallerstein, Immanuel, ed. 1964. *The Road to Independence: Ghana and the Ivory Coast.* Paris: Mouton.

Washington, Harriet A. 2006. *Medical Apartheid: The Dark History of Medical Experimentation on Black Americans from Colonial Times to the Present.* New York: Harlem Moon Books.

Watney, Simon. 1994. *Practices of Freedom: Selected Writings on HIV/AIDS.* Durham, N.C.: Duke University Press.

Watts, Sheldon. 1997. *Epidemics and History: Disease, Power and Imperialism.* New Haven, Conn.: Yale University Press.

Webb, Douglas. 1997. *HIV and AIDS in Africa.* London: Pluto Press.

Weiskel, Timothy C. 1980. *French Colonial Rule and the Baulé Peoples: Resistance and Collaboration 1889–1911.* Oxford: Clarendon Press.

Wendland, Claire L. 2008. "Research, Therapy, and Bioethical Hegemony: The Controversy over Perinatal AZT Trials in Africa." *African Studies Review* 51, no. 3, 1–23.

Wiktor, S. Z., I. Ikpini, J. M. Karon, J. Nkengason, C. Maurice, S. T. Severin, T. H. Roels et al. 1999. "Short-Course Oral Zidovudine for Prevention of Mother-to-Child Transmission of HIV-1 in Abidjan, Côte-d'Ivoire: A Randomised Trial." *Lancet* 35, no. 6, 781–85.

Wittrock, Björn. 2000. "Modernity: One, None or Many? Europeans Origins and Modernity as a Global Condition." *Daedalus* 129, no. 1, 31–60.

Wondji, Christophe. 1972. "La fièvre jaune à Grand-Bassam (1899–1903)." *Revue française d'histoire d'outre-mer* 59, no. 215, 205–39.

———. 1976. "Bingerville, naissance d'une capitale." *Cahiers d'études africaines* 16, nos. 61–62, 83–102.

———. 1982. "Quelques caractéristiques des résistances populaires en Afrique noire, 1900–1931." *Études africaines offertes à Henri Brunschwig,* Henri Brunschwig and Jan Vansina, eds., 341–58. Paris: Éditions de l'École des hautes études en Sciences sociales.

Wooten, Stephen R. 1993. "Colonial Administration and the Ethnography of the Family in the French Soudan." *Cahiers d'études africaines* 33, no. 131, 419–46.

World Bank. 1996. *Poverty in Côte-d'Ivoire: A Framework for Action.* Confidential report number 15640-IVC. Washington: World Bank, Human Development 3/Africa Region.

Yapi-Diahou, Alphonse. 1994. "Les politiques urbaines en Côte-d'Ivoire et leurs impacts sur l'habitat non planifié précaire: L'exemple de l'agglomération d'Abidjan." PhD diss., Université de Paris 8 Saint-Denis.

Zan, Semi-Bi. 1976. "L'infrastructure routière et ferroviaire coloniale, source de mutations sociales et psychologiques: Le cas de la Côte-d'Ivoire, 1900–1940." *Cahiers d'études africaines* 16, nos. 61–62, 147–58.

Zarwan, John. 1976. "The Xhosa Cattle Killings, 1856–57." *Cahiers d'études africaines* 16, nos. 63–64, 519–39.

Zola, Irving. 1972. "Medicine as an Institution of Social Control." *Sociological Review* 20, 487–504.

Zolberg, Aristide. 1964. *One-Party Government in the Ivory Coast.* Princeton: Princeton University Press.

ACT-UP: in Abidjan, 80, 102; in Paris, 107
administrative technologies, 86, 113,
    121–22
African labor: *apprentis* (fare-collectors)
    and, 150–52; colonial reliance on, 119–
    21, 127, 177; security guards and, 153–54
AIDS/HIV: Abidjan AIDS clinic, 5, 103,
    111–12; biopolitics of, 113, 133–34, 202
    n. 1; denial and, 1, 20, 26–27, 85; dis-
    crimination and, 24; educational ma-
    terial, 19–20, 161; epidemic of, in North
    America, 25–26; epidemiological statis-
    tics of, 179–80, 191 n. 6; ethnographic
    studies of, 189 n. 2; "exceptionalism"
    and, 6–7, 13, 176, 185–87; funding for
    prevention and treatment of, 8, 23, 36,
    41, 79–81, 202 n. 3; marches and, 79, 195
    n. 16; as a matter of life and death, 15,
    33, 85, 87, 89, 184; Montreal AIDS clinic,
    2–3, 90, 197 n. 9; international AIDS
    conferences, 3, 79, 89; life expectancy
    and, 90–91; politics of, 6, 13, 156, 175;
    prevalence of, in West Africa, 18; preva-
    lence of, in young girls, 200 n. 11; pro-
    liferation of words about, 184; religion
    and, 71–72, 86, 195 n. 12; resource flows
    for targeting, 202 n. 6; self-help and, 7,
    77, 83–84, 86–87; "talking groups" and,
    60, 84, 96, 98–99 (*see also* workshops);
    telephone help line and, 45–48, 50, 58,
    152. *See also* activism; prevention; testi-
    monials; treatment
anticolonial politics, 65
ARVs (antiretrovirals): access to, 5, 85,
    97–99, 106–8; businesses profiting
    from, 183–84; efficacy of, in early treat-
    ments, 4, 48, 89–90, 197 n. 10; funding
    for, 203 n. 6; high costs associated with,
    19, 102–3, 106, 108, 178–79; highly active
    antiretroviral therapy (HAART) and,
    90, 104; increased appetite as a side

effect of, 182–83; monitoring patient
    results from, 106, 179–80, 186; for pre-
    vention of mother-to-child transmis-
    sion, 93; resistance to, 105–6, 176–77,
    182; subsidized treatments and, 83, 97;
    triage system for distribution of, 109,
    174–75, 185; UNAIDS initiative to supply,
    101–5
Augé, Marc, 194 n. 3
AZT (azidothymidine), 2–3; for preven-
    tion of mother-to-child transmission,
    37, 93–94, 178, 180

Baoulé people: as a dominant ethnicity,
    122–25, 172; kinship structure of, 152,
    198 n. 15
Bédié regime, 165–66, 172; coup of, 169–71
Bété people, 152, 201 n. 17
Bingerville, 115, 126
biological citizenship, 108–9, 196 n. 2
biological difference, 104–5, 113, 120, 176
biomedical citizenship, 197 n. 11
biomedicine, 25–26, 177, 192 n. 14; AIDS
    activism and, 91, 106; in French colo-
    nial West Africa, 113, 117, 120–21
biopower: as defined by Foucault, 112–13;
    in French colonial West Africa, 113–14,
    133–34
bioracial differentiation, 116–17, 121,
    133–34
"biosociality," 178
biotribalism, 177
bisexuality, 162–63
Burkina Faso: AIDS relief efforts in, 16,
    183; clinical trials in, 37, 93–94, 108;
    epidemic prevalence in, 18, 20, 191 n. 6;
    government of, 192 n. 20; HIV testimo-
    nials and, 24, 31; HIV testing in, 20–21,
    191 n. 6; public health system in, 20. *See
    also* Ouagadougou (Burkina Faso)
Bush, George W., 179, 184, 202 n. 3

Marais, Hein, 85
Marie, Alain, 147
Marxist anthropology, 194 n. 3
medicalization, 25, 42, 192 n. 14
Merck's "028" study (1997), 92
miasma theory, 116–17
mistresses, 158–59
Mitchell, J. Clyde, 67
Montreal General Hospital AIDS clinic,
    2–3, 90, 197 n. 9
moral economy, 23, 191 n. 10, 200 n. 12;
    corruption of, 31, 59; as defined by
    Thompson, 22; of secrecy and milieu,
    164–65, 168, 173; self-help model and,
    8, 83–84
mother-to-child transmission of HIV, 37,
    77, 93, 178, 196 n. 3

National AIDS Committee, 29, 182
National AIDS Research Agency (ANRS),
    93
Newell, Sasha, 23, 200 n. 12
NGOs (nongovernmental organizations):
    ACT-UP and, 80, 102, 107; as advocates
    for access to HIV treatment, 107, 187;
    AIDS intervention efforts by, 40–41,
    74–75, 180, 202 n. 3; biopower and, 113–
    14. See also *Jeunes sans frontières*
Nigeria, 153, 191 n. 10, 195 n. 17
non-HIV diseases, 181. *See also* malaria;
    tuberculosis
North America: AIDS epidemic in, 25–26,
    48; early HIV clinical trials in, 89–92

Oil Shock (1970s), 7, 139
Ouagadougou (Burkina Faso): AIDS
    groups in, 57, 97, 182; culture of, 17, 30;
    L'Observateur Paalga testimonial in,
    27–28. *See also* Burkina Faso
Ouattara, Alassane Dramane, 169, 171
Oupoh, Joséphine, 195 n. 17

Pandolfi, Mariella, 6
parallel economy, 148, 155, 159, 162–63,
    200 n. 12
Parti démocratique de Côte-d'Ivoire
    (PDCI), 65
Pasteurianism: health practices in colo-
    nial Africa and, 119–21; Pasteur's ideas,
    116–18, 198 nn. 7–8; tropical Pasteur
    institutes, 118
"patient zero," 2
Péducasse, Virginie, 71, 74
pharmaceuticals industry, 25, 91–92, 101–
    2, 107–8, 184
Plateau, 168, 169; segregationist geography
    of, 116–17
Positive Nation, 81–83, 112, 161, 184
postcolonialism: housing policy and,
    130–33, 143–44; loans and debts and,
    140–41; mimicry and, 78; plantation
    economy and, 139–40; poverty and,
    141–43; struggles for sovereignty and,
    7, 11, 137–38, 187; technologies and, 176.
    See also colonialism; economic crisis
President's Emergency Program for AIDS
    Relief (PEPFAR), 179–80, 202 nn. 3–4
prevention: education campaigns for, 25,
    28, 70, 76–77, 160–61; of mother-to-
    child transmission, 37, 77, 93, 178, 196
    n. 3; resource scarcity and, 107, 183,
    185
prevention of mother-to-child transmis-
    sion (PMTCT), 37, 77, 93, 178, 196 n. 3
prophetic movements: ethnographic
    studies of, 194 n. 3, 194 n. 6; of Harris,
    64–65, 68, 85–86, 110; Soldiers of God
    and, 9, 71–74, 86
prostitution or sex workers, 113, 156, 162,
    190 n. 5

racism, 24, 176, 191 n. 12; bioracial differ-
    entiation and, 116–17, 121, 133–34

railway workers' strike (1938), 127, 137
religion: AIDS and, 193 n. 11, 195 n. 12;
  Catholicism, 52–57; Christian confession, 39
religious movements, 64–65. *See also* prophetic movements

"sanitation syndrome," 116–17
Scheper-Hughes, Nancy, 85
Schmitt, Carl, 6–7, 176, 196 n. 8
schooling, 145–47
segregationist policies, 11, 116–17, 134
self-disclosure technologies, 96, 101.
  See also confessional technologies or
  disclosures
self-help: groups for, 59, 91, 95–96, 99,
  156, 177; international organizations
  as advocates for, 7–8, 75, 82–84; Light
  for AIDS goal of, 77; moral economy
  and, 8, 83–84; Western assumptions
  of, 15, 86
sexual abuse, 167
sexual identity, 162–64, 168, 201 n. 4
sexuality: in Abidjan culture, 158–61;
  bisexuality, 162–63; disclosures about,
  157; mistresses and, 158–59; secrets and
  rumours of, 163–65; sexual liberalism
  and, 12, 158–59; sex workers and, 113,
  156, 162, 190 n. 5; transvestites and, 165;
  as a truth or moral barometer, 173; of
  urban youth, 18. *See also* homosexuality
sexually transmitted diseases, 146–47, 156,
  173, 191 n. 5, 191 n. 7
Skinner, Elliott, 69
social inequality, 143, 145, 156, 191 n. 5
social marketing programs, 21, 191 n. 8
social technologies, 85
*Société immobilière d'habitation de Côte-
  d'Ivoire* (SIHCI), 127–28, 131
Soir-Info (Abidjan), 165
Soldiers of God: administration of

prophecies and, 9, 72–75, 86; interviews
  with Queen of Mothers and, 71–72
solidarity: international organizations'
  efforts to foster, 7, 83, 87; *Jeunes sans
  frontières*'s mission of, 84; moral economy and, 8, 10, 84, 173–74; pragmatic,
  86; through testimonials, 9, 61, 71,
  74–75, 157; therapeutic, 96
structural adjustment policies, 140–41,
  155, 190 n. 2
structuralist economists, 139
Swanson, Maynard W., 116
systematic classification, 114, 121–22,
  133–34, 171

"talking groups," 60, 84, 96, 98–99. *See
  also* workshops
technologies of persuasion, 155, 157
technologies of the self, 12, 75, 84, 114, 174,
  176; as defined by Foucault, 8–9, 39;
  self-transformation and, 62, 66, 74, 110,
  138, 156
testimonials: charismatic, 9, 99–100; as
  commodities, 59, 157; fears and risks
  associated with, 84; first African public testimonials, 21–24, 173; to foster
  solidarity, 83–84, 109, 174; genealogy
  of public testimonials, 24–27; of Harris, 62–65, 68, 85–86; as indicators of
  success for AIDS programs, 8, 75, 31–33;
  Ouagadougou testimonials, 27–33, 59,
  173–74; religion and healing and, 71–75;
  self-development and, 60–61, 66, 68;
  social outcomes and consequences of,
  75–77, 86–87; at workshops, 41–44, 78;
  World Bank funding for, 79
T4 cell count, 95, 97, 196 n. 6
The AIDS Support Organization (TASO),
  20, 76
therapeutic citizenship, 9, 89, 110, 134, 186;
  and "biosociality," 177–78; clinical trial

Vinh-Kim Nguyen is an HIV physician at the Clinique médicale l'Actuel in Mon-tréal and the Centre hospitalier de l'Université de Montréal. He also practices in the Emergency Department at Montreal's Jewish General Hospital. He is an associate professor in the Department of Social and Preventive Medicine at the University of Montreal. He is the author, with Margaret Lock, of *An Anthropology of Biomedicine* and also the editor, with Jennifer Klot, of *The Fourth Wave: Violence, Gender, Culture, and HIV in the 21st Century.*

Library of Congress Cataloging-in-Publication Data
Nguyen, Vinh-Kim.
The republic of therapy : triage and sovereignty in West Africa's time of AIDS /
Vinh-Kim Nguyen.
p. cm.—(Body, commodity, text)
Includes bibliographical references and index.
ISBN 978-0-8223-4862-7 (cloth : alk. paper)
ISBN 978-0-8223-4874-0 (pbk. : alk. paper)
1. AIDS (Disease)—Africa, West. 2. HIV infections—Africa, West.
3. Medical anthropology. I. Title. II. Series: Body, commodity, text.
RA643.86.A358N489 2010
362.196′979200966—dc22   2010022501